You are not Crazy, It's your Hormones!

Why you gain weight, get cellulite, suffer menopause, PMS and other concerning health changes.

By

Brian Sher • Dr Robert Goldman • Belinda Orgo

DISCLAIMER

Please note that medicine is referred to in this book as the 'practise of medicine' because it requires constant re-education and re-evaluation to maintain proficiency and accuracy. The data presented in this book includes research on anti-ageing therapeutics written by the best and brightest minds and published by some of the most authoritative texts and journals in the world. But in less than five years from now, we will know twice as much about anti-ageing medicine and biomedical technology as we do today 10 years from now we will have more than five times the knowledge of this subject.

Because of the ever-expanding knowledge of medicine, the most any author can hope to do is to wisely and prudently put forth theory and practice as best as it is currently known. In preparation of this text, the editorial staff reviewed scores of published reports, hundreds of books interviewed many of the world's leading anti-ageing researchers and scientists. However, do not assume the material in this book is 100 per cent correct.

This book is not intended to provide medical advice, nor is it to be used as a substitute for advice from your own physician. At best, this book is meant to be an educational resource to guide your personal quest toward enhanced health and longevity. If you wish to initiate any of the programs or therapies described in this book, you must consult and work in partnership with a knowledgeable physician to do so.

Published by
REDWOOD PUBLISHING
Suite 1102 1 Newland Street
Bondi Junction NSW 2022
info@redwoodnhrt.com.au

First published 2004

You're Not Crazy, It's Your Hormones!

ISBN 0-9587281-2-7

Cover by Cherry Design
Typeset by Chapter 8 Pty Ltd

CONTENTS

ABOUT THE AUTHORS

Brian Sher

Educated at the University of New South Wales, Brian is one of Australia's most successful publishers, entrepreneurs, authors and speakers. Director and founder of Australia's first preventative medicine and anti-ageing clinic, he has been a consultant to more than 1000 businesses and is a sought-after coach. His recent book What Rich People Know and Desperately Want to Keep a Secret is an Australian best seller now published in 15 countries and translated into 9 different languages.

Dr Robert Goldman

Along with being a scientist, surgeon, inventor, researcher, entrepreneur and author, Robert is a former world champion strength athlete, holding more than 20 world records. He is recognised as a world expert on drug testing and anabolic steroids and has helped establish international standards in those areas. He has been awarded many patents for his inventions and is a co-founder along with Dr Ronald Klatz of the American Academy of Anti-Ageing Medicine and is Chairman of the Board and the founder and President of the National Academy of Sports Medicine.

Dr. Goldman has spearheaded the development of numerous

international medical organisations and corporations. A physician and surgeon with a second doctorate in steroid biochemistry, Dr. Goldman has served as an Affiliate Faculty/Visiting Lecturer - Philosophy of Education Research Center, Graduate School of Education, Harvard University and is a Senior Fellow/Visiting Lecturer - Lincoln Filene Center, Tufts University and Clinical Assistant Professor of Medicine at Oklahoma State University's Department of Internal Medicine. He is a Fellow of the American Academy of Sports Physicians and a Board Diplomat in Sports Medicine and Anti-Aging Medicine. He co-founded and serves as Chairman of the Board of Life Science Holdings, which is a biomedical research company with over 150 medical patents under development in the areas of brain resuscitation, trauma and emergency medicine, organ transplant and blood preservation technologies. He has overseen cooperative research agreement development programs in conjunction with such prominent institutions as the American National Red Cross, NASA, the Department of Defence and the FDA's Center for Devices & Radiological Health.

As an inventor Dr. Goldman was awarded the 'Gold Medal for Science' (1993), the 'Grand Prize for Medicine' (1994), the 'Humanitarian Award' (1995) and the 'Business Development Award' (1996). He has served as Chairman of the International Medical Commission overseeing sports medicine committees in over 176 nations and serves as a Special Adviser to the President's Council on Physical Fitness & Sports. Aside from the numerous books he has authored, he has also published over 200 articles and appeared on hundreds of national and international media presentations.

Belinda Orgo

Joined the Health Industry in 1997, first working in the fitness industry, then progressing into the anti-ageing and preventative medicine industry. Through her exposure to thousands of women with ongoing health concerns and her own personal experiences with PCOS (Polycystic Ovarian Syndrome), Belinda developed a personal interest in hormones and their dramatic effect on health.

This book is a demonstration of her compassion and dedication to empower women through knowledge. She has commenced and run seminars for doctors around Australia and New Zealand helping educate them on the use of hormone supplementation and application of biological replacement and the effect of this on restoring optimal health.

*"No matter what your age or gender,
restoring your hormones to their optimum levels
has the same effect as giving water to a dying plant"*

FOREWORD

by Dr Robert Goldman

Chairman of American Academy of Anti-Ageing Medicine

"You are not crazy, It's your hormones!" is an important and timely book for women and men. It will help you finally understand that many of the worsening health issues you face are not your fault and not something you can fix by changing your attitude or willpower, as many women are forced to believe.

For years the medical community, has led women astray. Unable to find answers to the many negative health changes that occur women have been frustrated or confused; their condition have even worsened as a result of wrong diagnoses or the lack of options or alternatives offered to them..

In seeking medical solutions to unexplained weight gain, depression, fatigue, irritability, muscle and joint pain, poor sleep and stress to name just a few, women have been told by their practitioner that they are crazy, lazy or that it's somehow their fault.

In most cases women are simply suffering a hormone imbalance brought on by a busy and stressful lifestyle.

This book addresses areas of medicine that are of critical importance and which are largely ignored or grossly mismanaged by conventional medicine.

Redwood has devoted extraordinary energy to the matter of education in preserving health and eliminating the debilitating symptoms of chronic disease and illness. The result is most commendable.

I thank them for taking the time to publish this book and encourage all people to learn, understand and practice the useful information provided.

WHICH HORMONES FOR WHAT?

	DHEA	Estrogen	Human Growth Hormone	Melatonin	Pregnenolone	Progesterone	Testosterone	Thyroid Extract
Overweight	✓	✓	✓			✓		✓
Low weight	✓	✓	✓				✓	✓
Skin	✓	✓	✓	✓			✓	✓
Hair	✓	✓	✓			✓	✓	✓
Joints	✓	✓	✓	✓	✓	✓	✓	✓
Bones	✓	✓	✓	✓		✓	✓	✓
Circulation	✓	✓	✓	✓		✓	✓	✓
Immune System	✓	✓	✓	✓				✓
Sex	✓	✓	✓	✓		✓	✓	✓
Sleep	✓	✓	✓	✓			✓	✓
Memory	✓	✓	✓	✓	✓	✓	✓	✓
Mood	✓	✓	✓	✓		✓	✓	✓
Stress	✓	✓	✓	✓			✓	✓
Energy	✓	✓	✓	✓			✓	✓

Part 1

YOU ARE NOT CRAZY, IT'S YOUR HORMONES!

Hormones have the most powerful influence on your body and on how you look and feel. They are the body's way of chemically communicating between the cells effectively telling them what to do. Your hormones affect virtually every function in your body. Your body relies on your hormones to go to sleep, to wake in the morning to help you get out of bed, to think clearly, to help you grow up, to maintain your health, weight and looks. They affect your mood, your ability to cope, your sexuality, your sexual drive, your ability to be fertile and reproduce, your skin, your hair, your eye sight, your body temperature...the list goes on.

In short they affect every thing we do. We all have them and without them we would simply die! From the minute we are born, our hormones play a major role in how we grow, age and function.

From the age of 25 we all begin to experience slow declines in our hormone production, causing a slowing down or decline in many of our normal bodily functions.

If your hormones are not functioning properly or are imbalanced or have been affected in any way, you will suffer some form of what modern medicine calls ageing or illness associated with ageing. Unfortunately many of us accept this as normal or inevitable. Some people accept the debilitating symptoms of hormone decline as an unavoidable way of life and are told by their doctors that this is normal for their age.

The good news is that this is not inevitable and you do not need to accept illness and loss of function due to ageing.

Women have gone to their doctors seeking answers for their concerns. Some common concerns are stress, fatigue and depression. Women have been told there is nothing wrong with them and to go home and take it easy. Doctors have sometimes prescribed women Prozac to help them with their nerves- effectively saying 'lady you are crazy'.

Millions of women have been misdiagnosed and have been prescribed some dangerous prescription drugs. In reality what they are suffering from is a simple hormonal imbalance, which has been brought about by stress and environmental exposure to drugs, alcohol and other environmental chemicals, poor nutrition, lack of exercise as well as natural hormone decline due to ageing.

Many of the complaints and concerns women have about their health, especially stress, fatigue and weight gain, can be addressed by first addressing their hormone imbalances with a skilled doctor.

THE MAGIC HORMONES

Here is just a short list of what our hormones are responsible for. Remember a decline in one or more hormones can cause a disruption to any of the body's normal functions below.

Functions of your hormones	Possible problems if your hormones are unbalanced
Controls our metabolism	Slow, tired weight gain
Controls blood sugar levels	Diabetes
Controls weight gain/loss	Too thin or too fat
Controls fat distribution	Unable to lose weight
Controls muscle mass	Unable to build muscle
Control body temperature	Too hot/too cold
Controls proper brain functioning	Poor memory
Controls sexual development	
Controls libido	Lack of interest in sex
Supports immune function	Frequent flu/ debilitating disease
Gives feminine qualities	
Relieves menopausal symptoms	Hot flushes, night sweats
Reduces the risk of heart disease	

Keeps joints healthy	Arthritis
Fights fatigue	Stress and tired
Improves memory	Poor memory
Increases physical endurance	Lack of energy and strength
Develops sexual desire	Disinterested in sex
Prevents depression	Depressed, anxious
Retards osteoporosis	Brittle bones
Improves skin elasticity	Wrinkled skin
Improves mood	Gloomy predisposition
Controls menstruation	Irregular painful periods

Our hormones are responsible for many critical functions of the body. They are the body's most important method of communication between the brain and the individual cells, as well as between the cells themselves. Therefore, we cannot function optimally when we experience a decline in our hormone levels.

This does not only affect 'old people'. Yet it is where we see the most obvious signs of our hormone levels declining. For example wrinkled or thinning skin, weak bones and muscles, loss of energy and vigour, loss of libido or sex drive, poor eyesight, frequent illness and disease, etc. It begins to affect us as early as our mid 20's where we can lose as much as 10-20% of our hormone production each decade following faster, in some cases, depending on how we treat our bodies.

If your goal is to stay young and healthy and to look good and feel great all through your life, you cannot ignore the information provided in this book. This will ensure your hormones are kept at your optimal level and you will feel comfortable and in control of your life.

More about this soon... first let's review the myths and politics that surround hormone replacement therapy.

THE FAILURE OF CONVENTIONAL MEDICINE

With the growing realisation of the inherent shortcomings of conventional medicine (treating the symptoms and not the cause), traditional medicine is facing the inevitable – the inability to cope with the ever-increasing volume and costs of treatment, as well as not providing any answers.

The scope and complexity of chronic medical conditions killing our society is astonishing – lupus, crohn's disease, chronic fatigue syndrome, osteoporosis, bowel cancer, prostate cancer, breast… cancer just to name a few. All too often the treatments proposed by conventional medicine are so "toxic" that they produce symptoms that are far worse than the illness. To test this theory all you have to do is ask someone who has been treated with pharmaceuticals for a long time for some of the above mentioned conditions.

In order to safely and effectively treat any illness it is crucial that you understand the underlying cause of the illness. Conventional medicine addresses the symptoms of disease. It does not address the underlying cause of illness and thus it is fighting a losing and frustrating battle.

HRT AND CANCER?

No wonder people are confused about hormones.

One day headlines in the newspapers praise HRT. They proclaim the effectiveness of HRT in treating heart disease, osteoporosis and Alzheimer's. The next day headlines are screaming that HRT may not benefit the above conditions and in fact may give you cancer!

The truth is that not all hormones are equal! Also not all hormones are used effectively by doctors to address the many diseases and conditions people suffer. Most physicians are not skilled in the use of hormones to address the many diseases we face. We will discuss the various types of hormones in a later chapter so you can understand the difference and know what to ask your doctor for.

WHAT ABOUT CANCER?

Despite the widespread use of synthetic hormone brands, such as, Premarin they have always been associated with cancer. The first cancer linked with synthetic hormone replacement therapy was cancer of the uterus lining (endometrium).

The recent resurfacing of the synthetic hormones and cancer association came from a government-sponsored study titled "The Women's Health Initiative" (WHI). This study was scheduled to last 8.5 years but was aborted at 5.2 years because the risks of using Premarin and Provera outweighed the benefits. Breast cancer was just one of the increased risks discovered. The study concluded that synthetic hormone replacement therapy DOES NOT protect your bones or your heart, two of the primary benefits once used by doctors as selling points to get women to fill their prescriptions.

The WHI involved large medical centres around the United States of America and was designed to provide information about the risks and benefits of conventional HRT. Half of the 16,608 women received conventional HRT in the form of Prempro (Premarin and Provera) and half received no active drug (placebo).

DESIRED OUTCOME:
The WHI hoped to achieve increases or decreases in breast cancer, stroke, pulmonary embolism, colorectal cancer, endometrial cancer, hip fracture and death due to any cause.

ACTUAL OUTCOME:
   The results were astonishing!
   29% increase in coronary heart disease
   41% increase in strokes
   22% increase in cardiovascular disease
   2100% increase in pulmonary embolism (i.e. lung blood clots)
   AND
   26% increase in BREAST CANCER

IMPLICATIONS:
The findings of the WHI were not news to many in the medical community. In fact many other studies had already shown the negative influences synthetic HRT had on cardiovascular disease, strokes, blood clots and cancer.

The information exposed by this study made international headlines. It made such an impact that it had physicians and patients questioning the safety and efficacy of these medications.

After all, Premarin and Provera had become such a prominent treatment for menopause and osteoporosis in our society.

WHAT CAN WOMEN DO NOW – SAFELY AND EFFECTIVELY!

Concern about the potentially life-threatening side effects of synthetic HRT caused many women to stop taking these medications. For many women this meant the return of hot flushes, restless nights, uncontrollable mood swings, no libido, crawling skin and crazy behavior.

DOCTORS SAY NATURAL HORMONES ARE BEST

Jonathan Wright, MD, categorically states "natural estrogen and natural progesterone (NP) provide all the benefits of the synthetic forms - and more - with many fewer side effects, while increasing your risk of endometrial or breast cancer very little, if at all!" He also says "when describing replacement hormones, the word 'natural' is used to refer to the structure of the hormone molecule, not its source." With this in mind, then, conjugated estrogen is really horse estrogen, not human; and medroxyprogesterone acetate (MPA) is a progestin and certainly not progesterone. The source for true, natural sex hormones is either the wild yam (Dioscorea composita) or soy. These are then biochemically converted to molecules identical to human hormones [Wright JR, NATURAL HORMONE REPLACEMENT 1996; p. 23.

Many women have already taken back control of their lives and are enjoying the benefits of safer, natural hormone supplementation therapy. If you are still suffering then read on, as you will learn how you too can take back control of your life.

HORMONES AND YOU!

Over one hundred different types of hormones pour into your bloodstream at a rate of billions of units per day. They are secreted by glands such as your pancreas, adrenal glands, pituitary gland, testes and ovaries then released into the bloodstream. Hormones then travel around activating, controlling and directing organs and tissues.

Hormones such as estrogen, progesterone, testosterone, pregnenolone, melatonin and DHEA make us men and women. Your hormones build bones, maintain muscle tone and protect your joints. They regulate your heartbeat and breathing. Hormones fight stress, calm anxiety, relieve depression and allow you to feel. They govern sex drive and fertility. They stimulate your brain and immune system and relieve pain. They govern the menstrual cycle and allow pregnancy.

Most of your hormones decline with age. All hormones in men and women decline when their endocrine glands cannot maintain the same production of hormones they did in their younger days. Noticeably, the decline in our hormones starts around our mid twenties and begins to bring on minor ailments from weight gain, loss of memory, loss of energy, loss of hair and loss of skin elasticity to major disability, deformity, pain, disease and sorrow.

The decline in the production of hormones and loss of energy, vitality and virility however is avoidable!

IF YOU ARE OVERWEIGHT, MENOPAUSAL, HAVE PMS OR CELLULITE...IT'S YOUR HORMONES.

As we have established the underlying cause of many chronic illnesses is hormonal imbalance. It is impossible to achieve optimal health without achieving and maintaining the balance of your hormonal system.

A hormone is a chemical substance produced in your body by your glands. They are a complex cascade of chemical keys that turn important metabolic locks in our cells, tissues and organs. All of our cells are influenced to some degree by these amazing hormonal keys. The turning of these locks stimulates activity within the cells of our brain, intestines, muscles, genital organs and skin. They determine the rate at which our cells burn up food substances and release energy and whether our cells should produce milk, hair, secretions, enzymes or some other metabolic product.

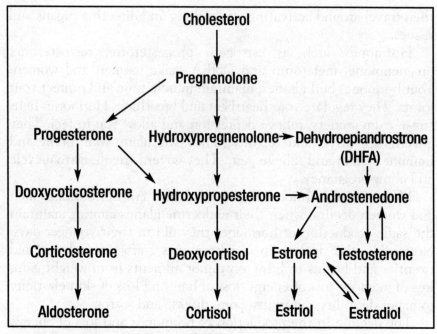

This diagram illustrates the pathways for hormones.
All other steroids are made from DHEA and Pregnenolone.

Your hormones are dependent on each other. They work as a team to maintain your health. If one is missing or insufficient, this will have implications on other hormones. Disease and health problems arise when members of the hormone team are not working at the same capacity as each other.

SYNTHETIC HORMONES = MONEY AND POLITICS

It would seem logical for you at this point to ask, "If there are hormones available that are natural to my body without the unwanted side effects of synthetic hormones then why do doctors prescribe synthetic hormones?"

The story of natural hormones is one of money and politics!

Natural hormones are bio-identical in structure to the hormones naturally found in your body. Bio-identical means that they are the exact same molecular structure as the hormones your body produces and may not be patented. A pharmaceutical company cannot own them exclusively. No patent means no money! No patent means that a pharmaceutical company cannot have the exclusive right to manufacture and profit from their product.

Tremendous investment goes into developing and studying a pharmaceutical product. It makes good business sense to protect their investment with an exclusive, patented product. Therefore there is little research and minimal marketing of natural hormones.

In order to sell a drug, a pharmaceutical manufacturer instructs physicians on how and when to prescribe it. Much of what physicians are taught after university comes from pharmaceutical companies that have done extensive research in order to justify a product. As no pharmaceutical company manufactures natural hormones, most doctors do not learn about them unless they do personal research. Research is often initiated by informed patients such as you. People like yourselves who have taken the time to learn, to ask questions and demand safer treatment options for you and your loved ones.

NO PATENT – NO PROFIT

Dr. Christiane Northrup, M.D., Assistant Clinical Professor of Obstetrics and Gynecology, University of Vermont College of Medicine, states: "Synthetic progestins, such as Provera®, Amen®, and Norlutate®, are made by taking naturalprogesterone from soybeans or yams and changing it chemically to compounds with progesterone-like activity that are not found naturally in your body... Another reason why natural hormones are chemically altered to synthetics is so that they can be patented by the drug companies who manufacture them. If a drug company cannot patent a drug, the drug company cannot make a substantial enough profit on it... But hormones that occur naturally in the body cannot be patented. They are considered generic and have been prescribed by physician for 50 years. Natural hormones have been used in Europe for decades. Women in the U.S. deserve the same" *(as do the rest of the world)*.

NATURAL IS BETTER THAN SYNTHETIC

Those who still wish to argue the case for synthetic HRT will usually be drug-company sponsored or have some vested interest in not advocating the switch to natural hormones. They will argue that there has not been enough research to provide evidence of the safety of natural hormones. This is comical, as these are the same people who know that synthetic hormones have been UNEQUIVOCALLY PROVEN to give patients cancer, stroke and deep vein thrombosis. Here they are saying that natural hormones may not be safe. No one has ever died of using natural hormones. Why? Because these hormones will not have any side effects if prescribed in the right dose by a skilled doctor. It makes perfect sense that these are safe and effective and there is science behind this because natural hormones have the same chemical structure as those produced by your own body. So, if you we going to get cancer or some other illness, you would get this anyway and it is not a result of your natural hormone supplementation.

In fact, studies show that natural hormone supplementation will save your life. One such study published in the New England Journal of Medicine, showed that men who died of heart disease all had chronically low levels of DHEA. More about DHEA later...

SO WHAT ARE NATURAL HORMONES?

A natural hormone is defined as a hormone that is biochemically and molecularly identical to the human hormone. It is derived from a plant.

When describing replacement hormones, the word "natural" is used to refer to the structure of the hormone molecule, not its source. When analysed biochemically, the molecules of estrogens, progesterone and other hormones produced from wild yam precursor molecules are found to be absolutely indistinguishable from those the human body produces itself. Thus, the crucial variable defining "natural" is not the origin of the hormone; rather it is the chemical structure.

Natural bio-identical hormones get their start from the wild yam plant (Diascorea composita). It is rich in "precursor" molecules and easily converted by biochemists into other molecules that are identical in every way to "natural" estrogens, progesterone, testosterone, DHEA and other hormones. These plant-derived bio-identical hormones are almost entirely without the side effects of the synthetic or semi-synthetic HRT drugs commonly prescribed.

WHERE DO NATURAL HORMONES COME FROM?

Natural hormones are substances that are produced from plants. They are structurally and chemically the same as the hormones produced in your body. The natural hormones we cover in this book include: estrogen (estrone, estradiol and estriol) progesterone, testosterone, pregnenolone, thyroid extract, melatonin and DHEA.

Synthetic hormones do not occur naturally in the body. They can be thought of as foreign substances to the body. No wonder they can give us so many problems! Synthetic patentable hormones like those found in Premarin, PremPro, Provera (medroxyprogesterone acetate) and methyltestosterone are artificial hormones that have been altered from the original hormone so they do not act or look like natural hormones.

Some patentable estrogens are derived from the urine of pregnant horses. Thus, the commercially available Premarin not only contains estrone in unnaturally high doses, but also contains many other hormones found only in horses. This is not natural to the human body. Other products such as Cenestin and Estratab are also derived from wild yam and soy plants. However, in some cases, the plant hormones are converted by biochemists to equine hormones similar to those in Premarin.

THE NATURAL HORMONE SOLUTION – BALANCE IS THE KEY

The goal of any natural hormone treatment should be to alleviate the symptoms caused by the natural decline in hormone production by the body and to bring the body back into hormonal balance.

Another goal of NHRT is to imitate the body's natural processes as much as possible, thereby eliminating most of the unwanted side effects and long-term risks of the traditional synthetic hormone replacement therapies.

The key to hormonal health is balance. Hormone treatment should be prescribed in the smallest effective dose in a plan carefully customised for you and supervised by a qualified physician who is knowledgeable in natural hormones. (Help with finding a doctor who will listen will be covered too!)

Natural hormone replacement therapy is the most effective treatment option not only for promoting optimal health but also for treating many chronic illnesses including: chronic fatigue syndrome, menopausal symptoms, heart disease, fibromyalgia, PMS, osteoporosis, thyroid disease and sexual dysfunction.

With the proper dose of natural hormones in combination with a supportive diet and vitamin and mineral supplementation you can retain your zeal and energy and achieve optimal health. You can also regain the youthful resilience that enables us to cope gracefully with the stresses that challenge us every day.

In the next section we will look at each of the natural hormones individually, although, it is important to note that the best outcome is achieved when they are used in combination.

Part 2

HORMONES FOR OPTIMAL HEALTH

Let's take a closer look at the benefits and functions of your eight optimal hormones.

- DHEA
- Estrogen
- Human Growth Hormone
- Melatonin
- Pregnenolone
- Progesterone
- Testosterone
- Thyroid Hormones

DHEA

DHEA (Dehydroepiandrosterone) is a steroid hormone. DHEA is produced by the adrenal glands (located just above the kidneys) as well as by the brain and the skin and is the most abundant naturally occurring hormone in the human body. In your lifetime you will secrete more DHEA than any other hormone.

Your DHEA level increases until around the age of 15. It then begins to drop off sharply so that at 65 you're producing only 10-20% of the DHEA that you produced at 20.

BENEFITS OF DHEA	
Enhances the immune system	Controlling alzheimer's, lupus, AIDS and chronic fatigue syndrome
Reduces the incidence of cancer, heart disease and osteoporosis	Effective in the treatment of autoimmune disorders
Assists in weight and fat loss	Improves liver functioning
Improves energy utilisation	Inhibits tumors
Lowers cholesterol, LDL & body fat	Reduces mortality, especially in men
Fights anxiety and depression	Increases libido in women
Relieves joint pain	Enhances memory

Often called "the mother of hormones" it is an androgenic hormone produced from cholesterol. The body uses it to produce the sex hormones of testosterone, estrogen and progesterone as well as cortisol.

When supplementing DHEA, 82% of women and 67% of men rated higher in their ability to cope with stress, their quality of sleep and general well being. DHEA has the ability to control some of the negative effects of cortisol. When the body is placed in a stressful situation, the adrenal glands respond by increasing the production of their hormones, including DHEA. This increase in production is essential in helping the body adjust to stressors such as infection, injury or illness.

Dr William Regelson at Virginia Commonwealth University agrees that if you want to maintain youthful levels of health you need to maintain youthful levels of DHEA.

LOW DHEA LINKED TO CANCER

Scientists now believe that a person's risk of cancer may be linked to their levels of DHEA. It has been shown that women who suffer from ovarian cancer have extremely low levels of DHEA, suggesting that this hormone helps to prevent this type of cancer.

One 20-year study found that DHEA levels were far lower in men who died of heart disease than in healthy men. Certainly, DHEA levels seem to be a predictor of coronary heart disease. A 1986 study published in the New England Journal of Medicine measured DHEA levels in 242 men aged 59-79. It was found that men whose DHEA levels were 140mcg or higher (20-year-old DHEA ranges 300-500mcg per decilitre) were less than half as likely to die of heart disease.

In a study of people with Alzheimer's disease, DHEA levels were found to be abnormally low. Many scientists believe DHEA may play a key role in improving functioning of the brain tissue and reducing the symptoms of Alzheimer's.

MENOPAUSE LINKS TO LOW DHEA

What researchers are now discovering is that menopause is also associated with low DHEA levels and subsequent reduced bone density in women. The ovaries produce their own DHEA and when this slows during menopause the adrenal glands cannot adequately take over. The resulting overall deficiency in DHEA may be why osteoporosis afflicts so many older women.

DIABETES LINKED TO LOW DHEA

While about 10% of diabetics suffer from low insulin levels, 90% suffer from insulin resistance. Their bodies manufacture normal levels of insulin, but they have difficulty using it.

As a result, insulin-resistant diabetics (with excess insulin in their blood) tend to have low DHEA levels. These low levels tend to contribute to heart problems and to obesity, particularly later in life. Insulin stimulates an enzyme, which destroys DHEA.

WEIGHT GAIN AND CHOLESTEROL LINKED TO LOW DHEA

In a 1988 study, DHEA was given to five men of normal weight at a dose of 1600mg per day. After 28 days of treatment, four out of five reported an average body fat decrease of 31% with no overall weight change. Their fat loss had been balanced by a gain in muscle mass. Simultaneously, their LDL cholesterol levels had dropped by 7.5%. This change in body fat to muscle ratio may be due to DHEA's ability to help expend energy rather than store it for further use.

In a study at the Institute of Hearmath in California, it was found that DHEA levels could be naturally increased by people practising stress management and by listening to relaxing music. The study showed a 100% increase in DHEA levels and a 23% decrease in the hormone cortisol (the stress hormone).

'THE PILL' DEPLETES DHEA

Oral contraceptives also have been shown to reduce DHEA levels. It has been suggested that women taking 'the pill' should consider DHEA replacement to negate its depleting effects.

Considering all the above evidence, it would seem logical that restoring DHEA levels and maintaining them at personal peak levels will help restore a biological condition of youth.

The peak DHEA levels for women range from 1,200-3000ng/ml and the peak DHEA levels for men range from 2,000-4,000ng/ml.

HOW MUCH DHEA?

5-150mg per day is a recommended dose of DHEA. It is best to start at the lower end of the spectrum and increase the dose as necessary so that you can accurately identify how much DHEA is right for you. Taking too much DHEA could cause your body's own production (as low as it is) to reduce.

The best way to take DHEA is transdermally - applied and absorbed through the skin by a cream containing the exact amount of DHEA you require. DHEA can also be taken in a capsule or troche form and is still tolerated by the body very well. You should discuss the best option for you with your doctor.

Your DHEA levels can be monitored through a blood test or a saliva test. You should have your DHEA levels checked every three months to six months to monitor your progress.

HOW CAN I GET DHEA?

Great news - fortunately there is no synthetic form of DHEA (yet), so you can only take the natural form.

In the US and some other countries, DHEA can be bought without prescription at the supermarket. In Australia, however, it remains a prescription only medication. You need to obtain a prescription from your physician and the DHEA will be individually prepared for you by a compounding pharmacy. This is good news because it ensures you will actually be taking the pure pharmaceutical grade of DHEA, which is not always the case in the over-the-counter preparations.

For more information visit: www.redwoodnhrt.com.au
or call 1300 304 638

ESTROGEN
(Estrone, Estradiol, Estriol)

Estrogen is one of the most powerful hormones in the human body and many are surprised to find that both women and men need estrogen.

Estrogen is what makes a woman, a woman. It is estrogen that gives women their softness, curves, breasts and helps regulate a woman's passage through menstruation, fertility and menopause.

Without estrogen men are infertile and may have a low libido. Men, however, are generally not treated with estrogen supplementation as it can cause prostate problems.

BENEFITS OF ESTROGEN	
Relieves menopausal symptoms	Develops sexual desire
Gives feminine qualities	Increases physical endurance
Controls menstruation	Improves memory
Improves mood	Fights fatigue
Improves skin elasticity	Reduces the risk of heart disease
Retards osteoporosis	Keeps joints healthy
Prevents depression	Supports immune function

If you are a woman with low estrogen levels you may experience fine wrinkles around the eyes and mouth, dry skin and hair, loss of libido, mood swings, hot flushes, loss of bone density, night sweats, vaginal dryness and itching, depression and painful periods.

Estrogen is not a single hormone. It is a group of 3 different but related hormones (estrone, estradiol, estriol) that perform functions that we normally attribute to "estrogen". Approximately 300 different tissues are equipped with estrogen receptors. This means that estrogen can affect a wide range of tissues and organs, including the brain, liver, bones and skin. The uterus, urinary tract, breasts and blood vessels also depend on estrogen to stay toned and flexible. It can be secreted directly from the ovaries or made in fat cells by conversion from DHEA.

The natural pattern of circulating estrogens in the human body is:
- E1 Estrone: 10-20%
- E2 Estradiol: 10-20%
- E3 Estriol: 60-80%

Estriol E3:
- Weakest of the three estrogens
- Readily converts to estradiol
- Levels increase following menopause giving the body some estrogen benefits

Thought to be anti-carcinogenic, it is the most protective estrogen against breast cancer. Research strongly suggests that estriol has less cancer-causing potential than estrone or estradiol and it may actually inhibit the carcinogenic activity of these other estrogen [Dr J Wright; Natural Hormone Replacement for women over 45].

E3 has been shown to actually inhibit breast cancer in mice. It has all the benefits of the stronger estrogens, but with fewer risks. It's only negative is that it's much weaker than other estrogens; hence more is needed to achieve the same results.

E3 has been shown to be clinically effective for the treatment of menopausal symptoms as well as postmenopausal symptoms and vaginal atrophy, dryness, vaginal infections, painful intercourse and various conditions of the urinary tract.

In women, estriol is produced in large quantities (together with progesterone) during pregnancy and it is the estrogen that is most beneficial to the vagina and cervical tissue.

High levels of estriol have been found in vegetarians and in Asian women who consistently appear to be at much less risk of breast cancer. Research has demonstrated that women with breast cancer have a reduced excretion of estriol.

Estradiol E2:
- Produced by the ovaries and is the principal estrogen found in a women's body.
- Relieves menopausal symptoms
- Protects against osteoporosis, heart disease and Alzheimer's

- Enhances mental acuity and memory
- Increases serotonin and endorphin levels

Estradiol is the most potent and is converted to the weaker estrone then to estriol when levels of progesterone rise. This is the hormone that protects against osteoporosis and heart disease.

It is also responsible for maturation of long bones, development of breasts, reproductive organs and secondary female characteristics. Excess levels of estradiol may be associated with adverse symptoms, including increased risks of breast and endometrial cancer.

Estrone E1:

The primary estrogenic hormone in the post-menopausal woman is made from peripheral conversion of androstenedione in adipose cells, liver and skin. It is also made from the conversion from estradiol. E1 is implicated in hormone-mediated cancers.

All estrogens (estrone, estradiol, estriol) occupy the same receptor sites. This family of estrogens works in concert with progesterone to nourish and support the growth and regeneration of the female reproductive tissues, as well as impart the characteristic female growth of body hair, breasts and distribution of body fat. It is important to realise that not all estrogens are equivalent in their action on breast tissue and may explain some of this controversy. Estrone is the most stimulating to breast tissue with estriol the least. Estriol has actually been shown to decrease the risk of breast cancer.

Synthetic estrogen replacement therapy, such as Premarin, however, seems to exclude estriol and are composed primarily of the other two and one that you don't even produce in your body! No wonder women have problems!

SYNTHETIC ESTROGEN	NATURAL ESTROGEN
Estrone 75-80%	Estrone 10-20%
Estradiol 5–19%	Estradiol 10-20%
Equilin 6-15%	E3 Estriol: 60-80%

THE ANTI-CANCER HORMONE

For more than 40 years physicians worldwide have been prescribing synthetic estrogen to women to combat the symptoms of menopause. Physicians continue to prescribe conventional estrogen replacement and women feel better as your body needs estrogen and the onset of menopause drastically reduces your production of estrogen. However, the WHI study has revealed the reasons why synthetic estrogen replacement is not the answer for women.

Estrogen therapy has come under controversy most notably for causing breast cancer. One study revealed patients on estrogen (with and without Progestin – synthetic progesterone) had a 30-40% increased risk of breast cancer. Another study, however, reported no increased risk of cancer. These conflicting results underscore the continued uncertainty over the role of estrogens in breast cancer. For this reason, estrogen treatment is not recommended for women with a high risk of breast cancer.

Women with breast cancer have been shown in one study to excrete 30-60% less estriol than non-cancer patients and higher remission rates of cancer occurred in those whose estriol levels rose. Therefore, low levels of estriol relative to estradiol and estrone correlate with an increased risk of breast cancer.

Synthetic estrogen therapy increases your chances of developing breast cancer. Synthetic hormone replacement therapy puts women at a higher risk of uterine, ovarian and breast cancer, along with all the undesirable side-effects.

The risk appears to be removed when using estriol in natural hormones. Couple this with the long-term benefits for your heart and bones and you've got a safe and effective treatment for menopause.

LOOKING AFTER YOUR BONES

The relationship between estrogen and osteoporosis has been studied intensively. A decline in estrogen, progesterone and testosterone causes bones to become thinner and more brittle.

Evidence suggests that estrogen replacement can help slow down osteoporosis but it will not reverse osteoporosis. Estrogen replacement does not build new bone but it can slow down the rate at which bone cells die.

HOW MUCH ESTROGEN?

It is important that you establish your estrogen levels with a saliva test or blood test. Using these results you and your doctor can work together to find out exactly how much estrogen you need. If your results show you have an estrogen deficiency supplementation of natural estrogen may be recommended and should be taken in conjunction with natural progesterone.

HOW CAN I GET NATURAL ESTROGEN?

You need to obtain a prescription from you physician and the estrogen will be individually prepared for you by a compounding pharmacy. This is good news because it ensures you will actually be taking the pure pharmaceutical grades of estrogen. The strength and combinations of the estrogens can be established by working closely with your doctor who should have a clear understanding of your family history.

Natural Estrogen combinations available include: E3, Biest and Triest.

E3 – (Estriol)

E3 is the safest of all estrogen replacement options. However, it is weaker than other estrogens, hence more is needed to achieve the same results.

BIEST – E3 (Estriol) and E2 (Estradiol)

Biest is the combination of two estrogens: estriol and estradiol. It is most commonly found in a ratio of 80:20, estriol to estradiol. This combination allows for all of the protection of estriol while providing the cardiovascular and osteoporosis benefits.

Biest (80% estriol and 20% estradiol) are becoming more popular due to concerns estrone may increase cancer risk. It is important for any woman with an intact uterus who is taking estrogen to also take natural progesterone to protect the uterus from hyperplasia (cell proliferation) and uterine cancer.

TRIEST – E3 (Estriol) and E2 (Estradiol) and E1 (Estrone)
Triest is the combination of three estrogens: estriol, estradiol and estrone. It is most commonly found in a ratio of 80:10:10, estriol, estradiol, estrone. This combination is very popular and contains all of the three major circulating estrogens. It is slightly weaker in its effect when compared to Biest. However, this can be compensated for by increasing the strength or by slightly changing the ratios.

For more information visit: <u>www.redwoodnhrt.com.au</u> or call 1300 304 638

HUMAN GROWTH HORMONE

Human Growth Hormone (HGH) is a hormone that is naturally present in the body when we are young, but tends to disappear as we age. People who have taken HGH have found it produces striking improvements in their health, energy and sense of wellbeing. The list of benefits just seems to grow.

BENEFITS OF HUMAN GROWTH HORMONE	
Decreases body fat	Provides energy and endurance
Enhances sexual potency	Improves immune function
Lowers blood pressure	Enhances muscle tone
Improves skin, bones and hair	Improves memory
Improves vision	Enhances ability to deal with stress
Enhances sleep	Is responsible for growth

HGH is a simple protein hormone released by the pituitary gland in the brain. It enters our bloodstream in bursts during sleep, particularly after midnight. It travels to the liver, where it is converted into a substance called insulin growth factor 1 (IGF1). IGF1 is the messenger molecule that travels to all parts of the body stimulating cell production and growth.

It is HGH that is responsible for telling our bodies to grow cells, bones, organs and muscles.

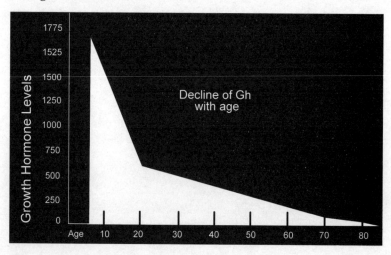

HGH is in plentiful supply until about age 20. Each decade from then on we lose approximately 20% of our HGH base level. So, by the time you're 60 or 70, your body has access to only 15-20% of the HGH you had in your youth.

HGH promotes growth by helping transport amino acids (the building blocks of protein) between cells and into cells. To create muscles and to build and restore organs, including the heart and skin, the body uses amino acids.

Low levels of HGH cause ageing because this hormone is primarily responsible for growth and regeneration of every cell in our bodies. If your body is deficient in growth hormone you will have limp, lifeless hair, drooping eyelids and cheeks, thin lips and obvious deep wrinkles on your face. Your mental state is also affected by increased negative attitude, fatigue, anxiety, depression and the need for more sleep.

Every day, regardless of our age, millions of cells die and millions more new cells are produced. When we are young and growing, the high level of HGH causes our bodies to produce more new cells than those that die off. Our bodies expand in size and look young and fit.

As we get older, less HGH is produced reversing the balance of new to old, more cells are dying than are being produced in every muscle, organ and part of our bodies. It's no wonder our body begins to break down. This is why we become less functional and begin to age.

Indeed, the correct HGH levels are the secret to maintaining youth.

Correct and specifically tailored exercise, diet, meditation, natural hormone treatment and nutritional supplements will all naturally increase HGH and prolong youth and vitality. There is little need to seek HGH supplementation unless you are truly deficient. But, from around 50-60 years, even those treatments are not enough. It is the firm belief of most knowledgeable physicians that to stay young many older people should supplement these treatments by taking HGH or IGF supplements directly.

The evidence supports them. More than 28,000 different studies on HGH indicate that human growth hormone supplementation is indeed one secret to maintaining youth.

The first great controlled, random, double-blind (and therefore super-accurate) clinical study in this area was undertaken by Dr Daniel Rudman at the Medical College of Wisconsin and was published in the prestigious New England Journal of Medicine in 1990.

Rudman treated 12 men aged 61 to 81 with HGH supplementation. The results were staggering. They actually reversed their body's ageing clocks.

Dr Rudman wrote: 'The effects of six months of human growth hormone on lean body mass and adipose-tissue mass were equivalent in magnitude to the changes incurred during 10-20 years of ageing.'

In interviews, the men reported incredible changes. One grey-haired 65-year-old found that his hair was turning black again. The wife of another man had trouble keeping up with her newly energised husband even though she was 15 years younger. A third man saw the wrinkles disappear on his face and hands.

Following up on his first test, Dr Rudman found that 26 other elderly men regrew their livers, spleens and muscles that had shrunk with age.

These tests opened the floodgates in the scientific world and subsequently thousands more tests have verified Rudman's initial results.

For instance, in 1992 medical researchers at the renowned Stanford University stated: 'It is possible that physiological hormone replacement might reverse or prevent some of the 'inevitable' sequelae of ageing.'

Dr Julian Whitaker, of the Whitaker Health Institute in California, has been prescribing HGH to his patients. In his view, HGH is most effective in combating the effects of chronic disease that involve muscle wasting, stroke, chronic heart disease and AIDS. He feels it can even be beneficial in treating burns and in helping patients recover from surgery.

Dr Bengt-Ake Bengtsson of Gothenberg, Sweden, states that the effects of 6 months of HGH therapy on lean body mass and fatty tissue was equivalent to reversing the ageing process by 10-20 years.

Dr Rudman does not believe HGH therapy will make people live longer, but that it will improve the quality of their life – stronger bones and muscles will improve mobility and independence mean fewer falls and broken bones.

In 1989 Dr Franco Salomon at St Thomas Hospital in London began testing HGH on adults who had their pituitary gland removed due to tumours. The experiment lasted 6 months, at the end of which patients had averaged a 12 pound gain in muscle and a 12 pound fat loss, with lower serum cholesterol.

Perhaps the largest HGH study on the effects of HGH treatment on humans has taken place at the Palm Springs Life Extension Institute under the direction of Dr. Edmund Chein, director of the Institute and his associate Dr. Leon Terry, a neuroendocrinologist from the Department of Neurology at the Medical College of Wisconsin.

Dr. Chein follows a HGH protocol that involves restoring HGH levels for patients who are deficient (IGF-1 less than 350 mg/ml) with low dose, high frequency HGH injections. Dr. Chein, by combining HGH injections with other natural hormones that are shown to be low, has developed a HGH program that he claims has been 100% effective for all of his patients. He guarantees that his patients will experience an increase in bone density of 1.5 - 2.5% every six months from the HGH treatment, as well as a loss of 10% body fat and an increase of 10% muscle mass. This HGH treatment protocol may continue until the patient attains the body composition of a twenty year old!

The following amazing results were published. The following figures were derived from randomly selected, self-assessments completed by 202 HGH patients between 1994 and 1996. In general, there were improvement from one to three months of starting therapy and they continued to improve after six months.

88% increase in muscle strength
81% increase in muscle size
72% improvement in body fat loss
81% improvement in exercise tolerance
83% improvement in exercise endurance
71% improvement in skin texture
68% improvement in skin thickness
71% improvement in skin elasticity
51% improvement on wrinkle disappearance
38% improvement towards new hair growth
55% improvement of healing old injuries
61% improvement of healing other injuries
71% improvement on healing capacity
53% improvement on back flexibility
73% improvement on resistance to common illness
75% improvement in sexual potency/frequency
62% improvement in the duration of penile erection
57% improvement on frequency of nighttime urination
58% improvement on hot flashes
38% improvement on menstrual cycle regulation
84% improvement in energy levels
67% improvement on emotional stability
78% improvement on attitude towards life
62% improvement in memory

L Cass Terry, M.D., Ph.D. and Edmund Chein, M.D, Medical College of Wisconsin and Palm Springs - Life Extension Institute.

HGH LIMITATIONS AND SIDE EFFECTS

HGH can only be prescribed by a doctor, under certain conditions. It has been reported to cause carpal tunnel syndrome and arthritis plus the growth of pre-cancerous cells. It has also been linked to water retention. Some men whose hormonal activity has been reawakened by HGH supplements find themselves growing small breasts. Finally, long-term HGH use in higher than physiological amounts, has been known to cause the enlargement of bones of the hand, head and feet.

However, HGH for anti-ageing purposes, is prescribed in small, regular doses to mimic the body's own natural secretions, which doctors have discovered cuts out most of the risks associated with its use in larger amounts. Recent studies have indicated that most, if not all, the undesirable side effects are reversed when the patient stops taking HGH or the doses are reduced.

Normally healthy young people under 30 should not be receiving HGH supplements. However, they should ensure their own production levels are kept at their maximum levels by implementing diet, exercise, vitamins and minerals and natural hormone supplementation.

IS IT EXPENSIVE?

Until recently, HGH supplements were difficult and expensive to make. HGH had to be extracted from the pituitary gland of human cadavers treatments were expensive. As a result, HGH supplements were used only in the treatment of dwarfism.

In 1980, two drug companies found inexpensive way to produce HGH in laboratories. However, it is still expensive and can cost $3,000-$8,000 per year depending on the dosage required.

Within the last 5 years the price has halved. These prices are expected to fall again soon, because the seven-year monopoly held by Eli Lilly expires. Together with recent innovations and such high demand from people looking to stay young this may drive the prices down further.

HGH replacement is also not desirable for all, as it can only be administered by injection.

AFFORDABLE ALTERNATIVES

People who wish to include HGH in to their prescription for healthy living, yet cannot afford it or are simply concerned about the needle have a few other options to stimulate their own production of human growth hormone.

HIGH INTENSITY EXERCISE – High-intensity exercise such as weight training, interval training, sprinting, squash etc. Long-distance running does not seem to be effective.

SECRETAGOGUES OR AMINO-ACID HGH RELEASERS – There are certain amino acids and nutrients, which in the right quantities and combinations can trigger the release of HGH. These are:

- Arginine
- Ornithine
- Niacin
- Tyrosine
- Glutathione
- Methionine

The amino acids need to be combined in the right ratios and taken simultaneously to achieve this outcome, however will be no where near as effective as genuine HGH, yet can cost up to 2/3 the price.

MELATONIN – Studies have also suggested that melatonin can increase the production of HGH (see melatonin next).

HOW CAN I GET HGH?

You need to obtain a prescription from your physician in order to obtain human growth hormone. The dose and frequency of injections needs to be discussed with a knowledgeable physician and must be closely monitored.

For more information visit: www.redwoodnhrt.com.au
or call 1300 304 638

MELATONIN

Melatonin is the hormone of sleep. The primary function of melatonin is to help you fall asleep, sleep soundly, dream and wake up in the morning. Melatonin is responsible for making you yawn and want to sleep and by activating the thyroid hormones; it wakes you up in the morning.

Melatonin is secreted from the pineal gland located in the brain. Very small amounts are also produced in the retina and gastro-intestinal tract. It is actually made from an amino acid called tryptophan. Tryptophan is then converted into serotonin. Serotonin is an important neurotransmitter associated with depression. Serotonin then converts to melatonin.

BENEFITS OF MELATONIN	
Increases quality of sleep	Is a potent anti-oxidant and captures damaging free radicals
Prevents jet lag	Improves mood and relives anxiety
Improves sleep disorders	Fights the growth of cancer calls
Improves immune system	Relaxes muscles and relieves tension

THE HORMONE OF SLEEP

Mysterious and at home in darkness, its cue is the daily cyclic variation in light. Melatonin production has a circadian rhythm - peak levels in the early morning and low levels in the afternoon. Melatonin is responsible for maintenance of our daily biological rhythm and its production is initiated by darkness, hence melatonin supplements should be taken at night. Levels peak between 0200 and 0400, but there is more to this hormone than sleep regulation. Melatonin also governs which other hormones are released.

Many of life's most common occurrences - job, travel, stress and ageing – can cause changes in sleep patterns and are likely to have adverse effects on melatonin secretion patterns. Identifying abnormal secretion patterns in late night samples can reveal sleep-wake cycle disturbances that result in fatigue and insomnia.

THE WONDER DRUG

Imagine a 'wonder drug' that extended your lifespan by 25% or more. Imagine, too, that this drug not only extended your life but maintained your youth, enabling you to enjoy work, sex and social activities with the same zest and vigour that marked your life in your twenties. Imagine, finally, that this drug had no harmful side effects or long-term dangers, because it is not actually a drug at all, but a substance that occurs naturally in your body.

The fact is, we don't have to imagine that at all. It already exists in every living substance from algae to humans. It is called melatonin.

Researchers at Tulane University School of Medicine in New Orleans have studies that suggest melatonin can stop or retard the advance of human breast cancer cells.

A 1995 study by an Italian researcher demonstrated that melatonin boosted the immune system of people under extreme stress.

Melatonin helps prevent heart disease by lowering blood cholesterol, combats AIDS, alzheimer's, parkinson's, asthma, diabetes and cataracts.

It has also been found to be effective in re-setting the biological clocks of travellers moving across time zones and is a natural sleeping pill inducing sleep without the side effects of sedatives.

In addition, it has been shown to be a powerful antioxidant that helps to keep the body young.

The main function of the pineal gland is to help govern our biological rhythms (circadian rhythms) that take place over the day, such as the sleep-wake cycle. It also governs seasonal rhythms. Researchers see this gland and hormone as a kind of orchestra conductor, coordinating and controlling our other hormone-release and immune responses. The pineal gland communicates with these other systems through its messenger, melatonin.

Changes in melatonin set off a range of responses, such as puberty, menstruation and sleep. It also alerts our bodies to produce antibodies to combat disease.

So, you can see how important the presence and maintenance of correct level of this hormone are for the optimal functioning of our bodies throughout our life.

As we've seen, nature isn't much interested in us after we've gotten too old to reproduce. Our pineal gland is our internal clock that 'knows' how old we are and when we are past our prime. It responds by producing lower levels of melatonin, signalling our other systems to break down, causing us to age.

What if we could somehow raise our levels of melatonin after they start to fall? What if for the rest of our lives we could duplicate the levels of melatonin we had in our youth? We would in effect be 'tricking' our bodies into believing they are still young, giving orders to produce higher levels of sex hormones and a well-functioning immune system to fight off disease ... chronologically we would be old, yet biologically we would still be young.

Researchers have found that melatonin supplementation helps the body mimic a youthful state. Not only that, but melatonin helps strengthen our immune systems, prevents cancer and improves sexual functioning.

One of the ways melatonin helps combat cancer is as a powerful antioxidant. It is the only antioxidant capable of penetrating every cell of the body and is the most active and effective of all naturally occurring compounds.

For example, in certain tests melatonin proved to be five times more powerful than glutathione and at least twice as effective as powerful Vitamin E. Furthermore, most antioxidants are either water-soluble or fat-soluble. Melatonin is making it a wider-ranging antioxidant than its vitamin or mineral counterparts.

HOW MUCH MELATONIN?

With melatonin, remember less is more. Although melatonin plays an extremely important role in our bodies, it is present in only tiny amounts, even at our youthful peak. Larger doses of melatonin won't help. With melatonin, remember less is more. Although melatonin plays an extremely important role in our bodies, it is present in only tiny amounts, even at our youthful peak. Larger doses of melatonin won't help. People with autoimmune disorders, leukemia or lymphoma should consult a physician before use. Melatonin could also interfere with fertility and pregnant or nursing mothers should also avoid melatonin. On the other hand women on HRT should take melatonin without fear of any ill effects.

As melatonin drops most sharply around age 45, melatonin supplementation should begin around then and not before, except for short-term use, such as jet lag. People with a family history of cancer or cardiovascular disease might begin in their late 30s. The idea is to start taking melatonin when your levels drop off and not before, because extra melatonin (above your optimal physiological needs) will not benefit you.

Remember, always take melatonin at bedtime as it generally makes you sleepy, so it should not be taken before you drive or operate machinery.

Remember, each person's physiology is unique so it is advisable to get your Melatonin level checked through a saliva test. Melatonin in the range 0.5mg - 12mg is usually effective. It's best to start on low doses such as 0.5 - 2mg and increase this if you find it does not help. Melatonin is best taken on an empty stomach 30 minutes to 2 hours before going to bed. Melatonin is effective in capsule form and also sublingual drops. You should reduce your doses if you find you are waking up tired and groggy.

HOW CAN I GET MELATONIN?

In the US and some other countries, melatonin can be bought without prescription at the supermarket. In Australia, however, it remains a prescription only medication. You need to obtain a prescription from your physician and the melatonin will be individually prepared for you by a compounding pharmacy. This is good news because it ensures you will actually be taking the pure pharmaceutical grade of melatonin, which is not always the case in the over-the-counter preparations just mentioned.

For more information visit: www.redwoodnhrt.com.au
or call 1300 304 638

PREGNENOLONE

Often referred to as the "parent hormone", pregnenolone is produced in the adrenal gland and in the brain from cholesterol. Pregnenolone is the precursor of all adrenal and sex hormones. Because of this if you do not have sufficient levels of pregnenolone you'll create a domino effect on all other hormones. The body can only produce desired amounts if your body has adequate amounts of cholesterol, vitamin A, thyroid hormone and enzymes. If these levels are insufficient, a low supply of pregnenolone will result.

Believed to be the most potent memory enhancer, it has also been shown to be beneficial in improving concentration, fighting mental fatigue and relieving severe joint pain and fatigue in arthritis.

BENEFITS OF PREGNENOLONE	
Precursor of many other hormones	Boosts immune system
Fights the effects of fatigue and stress	Protects against coronary artery disease
Relieves arthritis pain	Improves mood and memory
Improves heart health	Essential to full brain function
Protects against Alzheimer's disease	Aids in skin rejuvenation
Assists in alleviating stress	

BRAIN FOOD

It is sometimes called "brain steroids," since the brain contains higher concentrations than other organs or the blood. Pregnenolone is the most abundant hormone in the brain. Pregnenolone's concentration is 75 times higher than in the blood. Low levels of pregnenolone will undoubtedly result in memory problems and poor concentration.

Brain concentrations of pregnenolone peak at around age thirty. At age 75, there is a 65% reduction in pregnenolone production in the body compared to levels at age 35, thereby increasing the need for supplemental pregnenolone as we age.

An article in the Proceedings of the National Academy of

Sciences (Nov. 6, 1995), describes pregnenolone as "the most potent memory enhancer yet found."

Pregnenolone is proving to be a particularly useful hormone treatment for memory, mood problems, fatigue and depression. Animal studies have shown benefit in memory in animals treated with pregnenolone.

Pregnenolone has been found to play an important role in the acquisition of knowledge and the long term memory of learned behavior. (DeWied 1976, 1977) In a study with rats by Flood et al. (1995), pregnenolone was found to enhance memory at doses far lower than doses required of other steroids or steroid precursors, including DHEA.

Some people find pregnenolone improves energy levels, vision, clarity of thinking, wellbeing and perhaps sexual enjoyment. Some women report lessening of hot flushes and premenstrual symptoms with the help of pregnenolone.

TIRED AND STRESSED

Low levels of pregnenolone ensure you will be vulnerable to stress and depression and at a high risk of chronic fatigue syndrome.

In the mid 1940s, several studies indicated that a daily dose of 50 mg of pregnenolone reduced fatigue and stress among factory workers, airline pilots and other subjects. (Pincus) Today, there are millions of people who suffer from stress and fatigue who may find relief with pregnenolone.

SAY NO TO ARTHRITIS

Studies have also indicated that pregnenolone may be beneficial for treating rheumatoid arthritis. Since it is a precursor to the production of cortisol in the body pregnenolone was used as early as the 1940s as a treatment for rheumatoid arthritis. In daily doses ranging from 50 mg to 700 mg, pregnenolone was found to be effective for this condition and to be much safer than the corticoids, salicylates and other drugs used as treatments at the time. Daily doses of pregnenolone above 200 mg appeared to be more effective than those below 200 mg. (Davidson)

Pregnenolone was used in the late 1940's to treat rheumatoid arthritis but fell into disuse when cortisone was discovered. Unfortunately, the toxic effects of cortisone are many and severe, classically involving daytime euphoria, insomnia, hot flushes at night and osteoporosis. In contrast, pregnenolone was never found to have adverse side effects and can be used to withdraw from cortisone therapy over a one-month period. Because pregnenolone has normalizing effects on the adrenal gland this withdrawal from cortisone can be accomplished without the development of "Addison's" disease symptoms.

HOW MUCH PREGNENOLONE?

10mg to 100 mg per day is the recommended dose for pregnenolone. It's best to start at the lower end of this spectrum and increase the dose as necessary so that you can accurately identify how much pregnenolone is right for you. Pregnenolone is generally always used in conjunction with other natural hormones.

DHEA has been observed to improve the efficacy of pregnenolone. However, since both DHEA and pregnenolone have some similar effects (however, they have differences too), you should lower your dose of DHEA when you go on pregnenolone. The lowering of the dose should be the same amount as the pregnenolone dose. Before you add pregnenolone, though, make sure you try it separately to see what kind of effects it has on each individual. Once you know how you react to DHEA and pregnenolone separately, you can then combine them.

Pregnenolone can be safely taken in cream, capsule or troche form. The best option for you should be discussed with your physician. Literature reviews have reported very few side effects in either animals or humans. Side effects observed include acne and drowsiness and can be corrected by lowering the dose.

Your pregnenolone levels can be monitored through a saliva test or a blood test. You should have your pregnenolone levels checked every three months to six months to monitor your progress.

HOW CAN I GET PREGNENOLONE?

In the US and some other countries, pregnenolone can be bought without prescription at the supermarket. In Australia, however, it remains a prescription only medication. You need to obtain a prescription from you physician and the pregnenolone will be individually prepared for you by a compounding pharmacy. This is good news because it ensures you will actually be taking the pure pharmaceutical grade of pregnenolone, which is not always the case in the over-the-counter preparations just mentioned.

For more information visit: www.redwwodnhrt.com.au
or call 1300 304 638

PROGESTERONE

Progesterone is one of the two main hormones produced in the ovaries. The other, of course, is estrogen. It is primarily produced in the second half of a woman's menstrual cycle and is the hormone responsible for the survival of the foetus in the case of pregnancy. Men also produce very tiny amounts from the testicles. Progesterone is also produced in small amounts in the adrenal glands in men and women where it acts as a precursor for other steroids.

BENEFITS OF PROGESTERONE	
Precursor of other sex hormones	Essential for pregnancy and the survival of foetus
Restores libido	Prevents PMS
Protects against fibrocystic breasts	Restores proper cell oxygen levels
Is a natural diuretic	Protects against endometrial cancer
Normalises zinc and copper levels	Helps protect against breast cancer
Is a natural antidepressant	Normalises blood clotting
Facilitates thyroid function	Normalise blood sugar levels
Stimulates cells (osteoblasts) for bone building	Improves energy, stamina and endurance

A deficiency in progesterone will produce painful, tender, swollen breasts, particularly prior to a period. Lacking progesterone will also produce anxiety, stress, irritability, headaches, a painful abdomen, aggression and extremely heavy periods. Weight gain, specifically in the lower half of the body, swollen hands and feet and excessive water retention are all signs of progesterone deficiency.

WARNING: PROGESTIN AND PROVERA IS NOT PROGESTERONE

Natural progesterone is made from a plant source and is an exact chemical copy of the progesterone produced in your body.

"Provera" and "Progestin" are synthetic chemical analogues similar to progesterone, but different enough to have some dramatic side effects. The progesterone molecule has been chemically altered in order to be patented and owned by the pharmaceutical company. Synthetic progesterone, such as Provera, is foreign to the body and has actually been shown to inhibit the biosynthesis of progesterone.

"According to Dr David G Williams, Progestin can cause abnormal menstrual flow or cessation, fluid retention, nausea, insomnia, jaundice, depression, fever, weight fluctuations, allergic reactions the development of male characteristics. Natural progesterone, on the other hand, has few side effects: occasionally it may cause a feeling of euphoria for some women, it may alter the timing of their menstrual cycles" (Stopping the Clock – Dr Robert Goldman pg 87).

Natural progesterone does NOT produce the severe side effects that synthetic progestins do, including the increased risk of cancer, abnormal menstrual flow, fluid retention, nausea depression, etc. Natural progesterone, in addition to enhancing fat breakdown and preventing blood clots, counteracts carbohydrate craving that may promote obesity and cardiovascular risk. In addition, progesterone can relieve menopausal symptoms like hot flushes, reverse osteoporosis and enhance mood and libido.

FOR A HEALTHY BABY

Progesterone is most dominant during pregnancy. The main job of progesterone is to prepare the uterus for the fertilised egg. Progesterone helps to soften the lining of the uterus and makes implantation of the fertilised egg easier. It is manufactured in massive quantities during pregnancy. Accelerated production starts in the fourth month or second trimester, 10-15 times more progesterone than before pregnancy. It is also responsible for maintenance of the uterus during pregnancy, helps prevent uterine contractions and aids in the preparation of the breasts for breast-feeding.

Natural progesterone is prescribed to women who are undergoing in-vitro fertilisation (IVF) and other methods. The natural progesterone is given to women following an egg transfer in certain types of fertilisation methods. Treatment for all women using progesterone supplements continues for at least fourteen days following ovulation.

Progesterone is also an important hormone in preventing miscarriage. Without adequate progesterone, the uterine lining will remain rigid, thereby, making pregnancy difficult to achieve. The lack of normal progesterone production by the ovaries in the second half of the menstrual cycle is called luteal phase defect. Women who have this defect either are unable to have their fertilised eggs implant in their uterine lining or, if the egg is implanted, it is so weak that miscarriage is a certain outcome.

To lessen the possibility of miscarriage, women who have a luteal phase defect use natural progesterone supplements after ovulation to help maximise the chance of carrying a pregnancy to full term.

If pregnancy occurs in a woman who is taking progesterone supplements, her doctor may decide to continue the treatment for another 8 to 10 weeks until the placenta manufactures sufficient progesterone itself to support the pregnancy.

PROGESTERONE – THE PARTNER OF ESTROGEN

Natural progesterone enhances the action of estrogen as these two hormones are meant to work together to maintain hormonal balance. Natural progesterone is very useful to balance excess estrogen in the case of premenstrual syndrome and estrogen dominance. (More about this in the "For The Women" section)

For example, treating endometriosis with synthetic estrogen, so widespread among doctors, is a grave error and a terrible injustice to women.

"Women on Menopause", by Ann Dickson and Nikki Henriques, reveals that unopposed estrogen was first linked in 1970 to "abnormal cell growth in the endometrium," resulting also in the possibility of endometrial cancer. Today, women need to be aware of the many other serious side effects when estrogen is administered alone and their progesterone levels are down, e.g.: nausea, anorexia, vomiting, headaches and fluid retention leading to weight gain. It is important; say the authors of this book, for women who have other physical disorders to avoid supplementation with only estrogen, for

it can exacerbate high blood pressure, diabetes, migraines and epilepsy. Natural progesterone has been found to be very beneficial in the prevention and treatment of endometriosis and polycystic sydrome.

Progesterone and estrogen levels naturally fluctuate during the menstrual cycle. However, if progesterone is too low or estrogen is too high, a woman will experience symptoms. Natural progesterone effectively relieves the uncomfortable symptoms of PMS and menopause.

Natural progesterone supplementation combined with the right nutrients give real protection not only against menopausal symptoms but other scourges of older women (and men) such as osteoporosis and heart disease.

PROGESTERONE BUILDS BONES

Progesterone can stop bone loss and even reverse already existing bone loss.

To reverse osteoporosis, Dr John Lee prescribes natural progesterone cream, a diet rich in vegetables and grains to serve as a source of calcium and magnesium for bone mineralization, mineral and vitamin supplements and modest exercise.

To measure the success of this regimen, Dr. Lee conducted a study of 100 postmenopausal women ages 38 to 83. Bone mineral density (a measure of osteoporosis) was monitored. Dr. Lee observed an increase in BMD of 15% (which indicates reversal of osteoporosis). Natural hormone replacement therapy produced relief of bone pain, increased physical activity, height stabilisation and fracture prevention. The benefits of progesterone were independent of age and time from menopause or estrogen use.

"Progesterone affects every tissue in our bodies (because) there are progesterone receptors everywhere. Clearly, women who have had their ovaries and uterus removed (especially before the expected time of menopause) should be taking both natural estrogen and progesterone to prevent osteoporosis, as well as atherosclerosis, premature mental decline possibly breast cancer" [Ibid., pp. 71-72].

DON'T FORGET THE MEN

Progesterone is made in men by the adrenal glands and testes. It is the primary precursor of our adrenal cortical hormones and testosterone. Men synthesise progesterone in amounts less than women do but it is still vital to the body.

When the level of testosterone decreases, the relative level of estradiol in a man increases. These gradual changes can lead to estrogen dominance. Estrogen dominance in men stimulates breast cell growth and prostate hypertrophy.

PROSTATE HEALTH

Estrogen dominance is responsible for the majority of breast cancers and is the only known cause of endometrial cancer in women. Since the male prostate is the embryonic equivalent of the uterus, it should not be surprising that estrogen dominance is also a major cause of prostate cancer. Research studies have shown that when prostate cells are exposed to estrogen, the cells can proliferate and become cancerous. When progesterone or testosterone was added, cancer cells die.

Natural progesterone is recommended for all men over 40 years of age or even earlier if there is a history of prostate cancer or BPH.

PROGESTERONE AND OSTEOPOROSIS

In Alternative Medicine: 'The definitive guidebook' a physician reports working with twelve men, all in their late seventies, who were suffering osteoporosis. The physician advised the men to systematically massage natural progesterone into their skin on a daily basis. All began to experience relief from their condition and reported that after three months, they were also experiencing an improved urine flow, with less pressure on their prostate glands and a noticeable decrease in nightly urination.

For those men who have already been chemically or surgically castrated for their prostate treatment and are at high risk of osteoporosis, Dr Lee has found that "if one wishes to prevent or treat the castration-induced osteoporosis, it is possible to safely supplement progesterone to replace testosterone in these men."

Dr Lee has pointed to research that suggests that too much progesterone in men can prevent sperm maturation possibly acting as a contraceptive. Progesterone does not cause feminising effects in men.

HOW MUCH PROGESTERONE?

You can measure your progesterone levels by a saliva or blood test. Since progesterone levels are apt to be highest two or three days after ovulation, it is wise to check hormone levels around day 18 to 21 of the menstrual month, counting day one as the first day of the preceding period.

Your progesterone levels are low during the first phase of your menstrual cycle (follicular phase). Levels increase sharply for a maximum of ten days following ovulation, which occurs around day 14. Levels decline rapidly at about 4 days prior to menstruation.

Once you and your physician have determined an appropriate dose, the best way to deliver this natural progesterone to the body is with a quality transdermal progesterone cream or in a troche.

Natural progesterone cream is one sure way of combating estrogen dominance and the symptoms of premenstrual syndrome without decreasing the natural amount occurring in the body. It is usually recommended daily, except the days of menses. The dose will depend on the severity of your symptoms.

For osteoporosis Dr John Lee recommends 5-20mg applied to the skin daily from days 12-24 in menstruating women or for 24-25 days of the calendar month in postmenopausal women.

Natural progesterone, 8mg to 40mg, is recommended for all men over 40 years of age or even earlier if there is a history of prostate cancer or BPH.

HOW CAN I GET PROGESTERONE?

Natural progesterone remains a prescription only medication in Australia. It is available in the US and some other countries without prescription at the supermarket. You need to obtain a prescription from your physician and a compounding pharmacy can individually prepare the strength you require.

PLEASE BE WARNED: A wild yam cream is NOT progesterone. Health food store wild yam formulations and over the counter pharmacy products are NOT progesterone. Wild yam cream contains phyto-estrogens which may increase the body's production of progesterone, but it, in itself is not a hormone or a precursor to a hormone. The truly therapeutic, pharmaceutical grade of natural progesterone can ONLY be supplied with a prescription by a compounding pharmacy.

For more information visit: <u>www.redwwodnhrt.com.au</u>
or call 1300 304 638

TESTOSTERONE

Testosterone is a powerful anabolic hormone produced by men and woman. Although women have testosterone levels one-tenth to one-twelfth the levels of men, it is important to realise its importance for both sexes.

In men, although the adrenal glands produce some testosterone, most of it is produced in the testicles. In women, the adrenal glands and ovaries produce testosterone and estrogen is manufactured directly from testosterone. This is why it is essential for a woman who has had a hysterectomy to use natural testosterone supplementation.

BENEFITS OF TESTOSTERONE	
Stimulates libido in men and women	Improves osteoporosis
Reduces body fat	Improves mood and depression
Improves muscle mass	Improves auto-immune disorders
Fights fatigue	Improves the symptoms of diabetes
Reduces the risk of heart disease	Helps in treatment of lupus

Testosterone is responsible for stimulating the libido in both sexes. Testosterone is necessary in men for erections, ejaculations and fertility. Women need testosterone for sexual desire and to maintain sensitivity in the nipples and clitoris.

But, it's not all about sex!

TESTOSTERONE LOWERS CHOLESTEROL

Testosterone protects the heart and arteries, reduces the risk of heart disease and counters high cholesterol.

Moller, a Danish physician, found that 83% of patients' experienced a significant decline in their cholesterol levels while supplementing their testosterone. Undoubtedly these patients would have felt much better on this therapy rather than on the conventional cholesterol-lowering medications which have debilitating side effects such as nausea, gall bladder disease, diminished libido, liver problems and abdominal pain.

BUILDS MUSCLE TONE – REDUCES CELLULITE

Testosterone builds muscle and improves muscle tone. It preserves bone mass and reduces fat and cellulite. It also prevents muscle and joint pain, osteoporosis in men, obesity.

Men diagnosed with hypogonadism are good candidates for testosterone replacement therapy (TRT).

One study of men over 50 who received TRT found that it renewed strength, improved balance, increased red blood cell count, increased libido and lowered LDL cholesterol.

Dr Michael Perring, medical director of Optimal Health Clinic in London, believes that TRT in conjunction with DHEA is beneficial to men with low testosterone levels. Numerous studies have also shown the link between low testosterone and high risks of cardiovascular disease.

Research suggests testosterone therapy in men may reverse prostate growth and PSA levels. PSA levels are the levels revealed from a blood test that when elevated may indicate an enlarged prostate gland or prostate cancer. Testosterone was found not only to reduce the PSA levels but also reverse the growth of the prostate gland. However, there is concern that testosterone could adversely affect the prostate cancer, therefore it is suggested that saw palmetto, DIM or indole 3 carbinol is taken with the testosterone to block any of the negative effects.

PROOF IT WORKS

Testosterone increases the bone mineral density of the spine and hip, fat-free mass, prostate volume, erythropoiesis, energy and sexual function [Journal of Clinical Metabolism, August 2000]

A recent study has shown that women with osteoporosis who took a combination of estrogen and testosterone increased their bone density. [Dr J Wright; Natural Hormone Replacement for Women over 45, pg 84]

In men, testosterone is produced in the testes, by a group of cells known as Leydig cells. These cells begin secreting high doses of testosterone during puberty to trigger increased lean muscle mass, sex organ growth, bone formation, deeper voice and higher energy levels. Peak testosterone levels are reached in a man's early to mid-20s.

As a man ages, the Leydig cells that secrete testosterone, begin to wear away. It is because of this, between the ages of 40 and 70, the average man loses nearly 60% of the testosterone inside his body. Other lifestyle factors, such as overtraining, stress and alcohol, can also hasten the deterioration of Leydig cells and cause testosterone levels to drastically decline.

Testosterone stimulates the body's development of muscle, bone, skin and sex organs, along with masculine physical features, such as hair growth. Scientists recently have discovered that testosterone also improves mental power, by enhancing visual and perceptual skills. Low levels can disrupt the body's blood sugar metabolism, leading to obesity and diabetes. Chronic deficiencies may also promote the early onset of osteoporosis and heart disease. Its use is popularly associated with enhancing libido but research is indicating that it is a vital factor in the prevention of cardiovascular disease as well as improving energy levels, bone density, muscle tone, prostate health, moods and vitality.

Men, if you feel fatigued day and night, are losing your self confidence and feel depressed, anxious or overly emotional, have constant restless sleeps, or are disinterested in sex and your memory is suffering, then this is a good indication that your testosterone levels are low.

HOW MUCH TESTOSTERONE?

Men, should you be considering natural testosterone replacement, it is important to undergo a full assessment through saliva and/or blood tests with your physician. You will need to have your prostate checked if you don't want to end up with more problems!

Women, you too will need to have your testosterone levels checked through a saliva and/or blood test.

Testosterone is best administered through a cream or a troche as it is well absorbed both transdermally through the skin and also through the membrane of the mouth using a troche.

The dosage needs to be appropriate to your test results and the objectives you are trying to achieve.

Doses for woman usually average from 2mg – 10mg per day and for men from 25mg – 200mg daily.

As with all other natural hormone treatments, the effects of testosterone must be monitored. Signs of too much testosterone treatment include; over-developed muscles, excess body odour, greasy hair, exaggerated aggression and disruptive sexual desire. If you experience any of these signs you should reduce the dose and consult your physician who can adjust the dose to a more suitable level.

HOW CAN I GET TESTOSTERONE?

Testosterone is a steroid hormone and therefore remains a prescription only medication. You need to obtain a prescription from you physician. The testosterone preparation that you and your physician have decided upon can be individually prepared for you by a compounding pharmacy. Having the preparation made by a compounding pharmacy ensures that you will actually be taking the pure pharmaceutical grade of testosterone.

For more information visit: www.redwoodnhrt.com.au

or call 1300 304 638

THYROID HORMONES

You may have a thyroid problem if you:

- Gain weight despite diet and exercise
- Are constipated most of the time
- Feel tired, run down and exhausted
- Feel cold, even when others are hot
- Have brittle hair or your hair is falling out
- Have nails that break easily and split
- Experience longer, heavier and more frequent periods
- Have dry, scaly skin
- Bruise easily
- Feel depressed
- Have trouble sleeping
- Have reduced interest in sex
- Have an increased sensitivity to light
- Have recurrent infections
- Suffer from headaches or migraine headaches

If you answered yes to six or more of these questions then you should investigate you thyroid function further.

Smooth functioning of the overall body chemistry depends on the health of your thyroid gland. Untreated thyroid disease leads to elevated cholesterol levels, heart disease, infertility, fatigue, muscle weakness, poor mental function, depression, weight gain and an increased risk of cancer. But first you need to understand how your thyroid works.

THE BUTTERFLY SHAPED GLAND

The thyroid is a butterfly shaped gland located in the lower part of the neck just below your "Adam's Apple". Thyroid function is very complex and exerts a profound effect on the function of nearly every other organ in the body. The thyroid affects all metabolic activity. It regulates temperature, heart rate and metabolism. If your thyroid isn't functioning optimally, neither are you.

Your thyroid increases fat breakdown resulting in weight loss as well as lowering cholesterol. Lowering your cholestrol helps protect

BENEFITS OF THYROID HORMONE	
Speeds up your metabolism	Helps control weight
Help keep skin soft and flexible	Provides a certain quickness of the mind
Prevents fatigue	Stimulates fat burning and dissolves cholesterol
Keeps you feeling young and healthy	Reduces the risk of heart disease
Prevents dry hair and hair loss	Reduces the risk of cancer
Protects the brain, heart and kidneys	Prevents memory and concentration problems
Protects the digestive and immune system	Boosts blood circulation, increasing supply of nutrients, oxygen, water and hormones to cells

against cardiovascular disease. It also relieves symptoms of thin sparse hair, dry skin and thin nails. People who suffer from low thyroid function tend to experience fatigue and low energy, slowness in their speech and actions, forgetfulness, mental confusion, depression, arthritis-like pain and susceptibility to colds and infections.

THE VERY COMPLICATED MADE EASY

The thyroid hormone works endlessly to combine tiny amounts of iodine with an amino acid called tyrosine in order to make thyroxin (T4) and triiodothyronine (T3). These hormones are responsible for converting calories and oxygen into energy for every cell of your body. 90% of the thyroid gland's production is made up of T4 and 10% is made up of T3. The pituitary gland also participates too, as it releases a hormone, appropriately named, thyroid-stimulating hormone (TSH) which stimulates the thyroid to release it's hormones.

Initially thyroid hormone is produced in the thyroid gland as a storage form of thyroid hormone called T4. Once in the body, this circulating T4 is converted to the active form of T3. As we age, the production of T4 diminishes. In addition, the conversion of T4 to the active form of T3 also diminishes, resulting in less stimulation of the cells.

Your body needs thyroid hormone to burn oxygen and produce ATP that is the fuel that runs the body. If your body is weakened due to an inadequate supply of thyroid hormone, you will not be able to burn up proper amounts of oxygen, thereby giving you less energy and symptoms of thyroid insufficiency. In addition, you will be unable to keep up mentally and physically as you once did. In addition, the immune system slows down, becoming weaker and less effective.

When the conversion of T4 to T3 doesn't occur, hypothyroidism (underactive thyroid) is a result.

THE UNDERACTIVE THYROID

Hypothyroidism (underactive thyroid) is the most common thyroid disorder and most commonly strikes after age 40. When you are unable to efficiently perform this conversion of T4 to T3 you may have hypothyroidism and your symptoms may include:

- Dry, pale skin
- Fatigue, lack of energy, lethargy, especially in the morning
- Cold hands and feet
- Depression, anxiety
- Low body temperature
- Weight gain or increased difficulty losing weight
- Decreased libido
- Headaches, migraines
- Irregular menstruation
- Chronic PMS
- Impaired memory and concentration
- Thinning hair
- Nails that are brittle and break easily
- Stiffness of the joints
- Muscle cramps and frequent muscle aches
- Fluid retention
- Irritability
- Intolerance to cold or heat
- Hair loss or dry hair
- Decreased heart rate
- Impaired hearing
- Dry skin and puffiness in the face, hands and feet
- Possible development of a goitre

IS YOUR THYROID MAKING YOU FAT?

As main regulators of the body's rate of metabolism, thyroid hormones have a profound impact on weight. By increasing enzyme levels that produce energy, thyroid hormones control how the body burns up carbohydrates and fats.

If the body and its metabolism are likened to an engine, thyroid hormone levels may be seen as setting the "speed" at which the engine "idles." These hormones accelerate the basal metabolic rate of most cells in the body. This is important, because a low resting metabolic rate has been cited as a strong risk factor for weight gain and obesity.

Hypothyroidism occurs when the thyroid gland does not produce enough "energy-generating" thyroid hormones. Weight gain is a classic symptom of this dysfunction. In such cases, levels of thyroid-stimulating hormone (TSH) may rise in an attempt to spur more production and secretion of thyroid hormones from the thyroid gland.

In addition, overweight women with a family history of obesity may have lower levels of T3 in their blood. Treatments to raise T3 levels may help reduce some metabolic risk factors associated with abdominal obesity in some overweight women. In a subset of these individuals, then, it may be a low T3/T4 ratio or a low T3/reverse T3 ratio, rather than a blanket deficiency of all thyroid hormones that sets the stage for weight gain.

Besides disrupting metabolism, thyroid imbalances may affect appetite control. Studies suggest that thyroid hormones may modulate levels of leptin, a hormone produced from fat cells that is believed to control hunger and stabilize energy levels which may play an important role in eating disorders and chronic obesity.

IS YOUR THYROID MAKING YOU CRAZY?

It is not uncommon for women with thyroid problems to suffer from depression. One explanation for this is that the most biologically active form of thyroid hormone, T3 is actually a bona fide neurotransmitter that regulates the action of serotonin, norepinephrine GABA (gamma amino-butyric acid), which are important for alleviating anxiety.

T3 is found in large quantities in the limbic system of the brain, the area that is important for emotions such as joy, panic, anger and fear. If you don't have enough T3, or if its action is blocked, an entire cascade of neurotransmitter abnormalities may ensue and can lead to mood and energy changes, including depression.

Hypothyroidism and depression are related on many levels. For instance, the neurotransmitter serotonin and thyroid hormone, both T3 and T4, are inextricably related in that the main building block that stabilises mood and anxiety. This means it is quite possible that low thyroid function can deplete your body of serotonin and other mood-stabilising neurotransmitters. It also means that chronic depression and sadness may deplete your body of tyrosine stores and T3, which is also necessary to maintain a healthy mood and energy.

Which comes first: the depression or the low thyroid? We suspect they occur simultaneously. While one does not cause the other, per se, it appears that similar emotional or behavioural patterns such as learned helplessness or not believing you can have your say may predispose you to both low thyroid and depression. Evidence of this is supported by the fact that, for many individuals, the depression and the thyroid have to be treated at the same time in order for thyroid function and mood to return to normal. But it can be a vicious cycle. Psychiatrists say that over time many patients who are treated for depression or anxiety with medications can eventually develop thyroid problems. No one knows why this is so (we suspect it is because antidepressants deplete neurotransmitter levels over time), but scientists are beginning to realise that thyroid disease is really a mind – body disease – its symptoms occur simultaneously in the mind (in the form of depression and lack of concentration) as well as in the body. This is why depression so often persists in women with thyroid disease; even after their thyroid hormone levels are corrected.

Research has now shown that improving thyroid levels will

alleviate many of the symptoms of thyroid insufficiency and allow our system to function more effectively and efficiently.

WHAT CAUSES A SICK THYROID?

SELENIUM DEFICIENCY - Selenium is necessary for the conversion of T4 to T3. (Incomplete conversion results in high levels of reverse T3, an inactive hormone.)

ESTROGEN DOMINANCE - Caused by stress and pollution. Estrogen suppresses thyroid function.

MERCURY – Mercury can contaminate the thyroid gland.

STRESS – Stress causes decreased adrenal gland function and prevents the thyroid gland from functioning optimally.

IF YOU THINK YOU HAVE HYPOTHYROIDISM

If you have a family history of hypothyroidism, fit the symptom profile for hypothyroidism as listed above, or suspect you have a thyroid problem here are some ideas to get you closer to a solution.

GIVE YOURSELF THE THYROID NECK-CHECK.

Hold a mirror in your hand and focus on the area of your neck just below the "Adam's Apple". Take a drink of water and swallow. As you swallow, look at your neck and check for any bulges or a protrusion in this area. If you see any bulges you should consult your physician.

HOW TO MONITOR YOUR BASAL BODY TEMPERATURE

One of the most sensitive tests for thyroid function can be done outside a lab. The basal body temperature test is an early morning temperature taken before getting out of bed and it is recommended that you do the morning temperature sampling for ten days in a row. Dr Broda Barnes formulated this test.

1. Upon waking in the morning, before you get out of bed, place the thermometer under your armpit

2. Record you temperature. It should be at least 36.5 degrees celsius. Any temperature less that this indicates thyroid insufficiency.

Menstruating women should start this ten-day period on the third day of their cycle. It is best to use a basal thermometer, as it is more accurate for this purpose than a digital electronic thermometer. Dr. Barnes also suggests that the thermometer not be used orally, but instead used under the arm, with the person lying quietly in bed, the arm resting comfortably at the side.

Dr. Barnes felt that this test was a check on the most basic function of the thyroid gland: its ability to regulate the metabolic furnace of the body to control temperature. An average of ten days is a very useful indication, therefore, of one's overall thyroid status in many people it may well be more accurate than the blood tests. Temperature testing however, is not infallible like any other test, it should never be used alone to rule in or rule out a thyroid condition, or to dictate therapy. This is simply a good piece of information that should be used wisely with your physician.

A low basal body temperature result, although it may be possibly due to low adrenal hormones, does warrant further investigation with thyroid panel blood tests.

GET A REAL MEDICAL DIAGNOSIS

If you think you may have an underactive thyroid, but have had the run of the mill TSH blood test with a "normal" result, you and a knowledgeable doctor may want to take a second look.

If you suspect you have an underactive thyroid, blood tests should not be limited to the "faithful" TSH blood test. This method is scientifically outdated and not all doctors are up to date. To get an accurate picture of what your thyroid hormones are doing you need to work with a physician who understands thyroid problems. You need to demand a full panel of tests, including TSH, free T4, free T3, reverse T3 and possibly thyroid anti-bodies. (These tests are considered a complete battery of thyroid function tests.)

PLEASE FIX MY THYROID!

If your tests indicate that you have a thyroid problem, you'll be presented with a variety of treatment and prescription medication options. The best option is to get the treatment that has the correct balance of both T4 and T3, the two hormones that you're trying to replace. Here are the current choices:

DIET – In hypothyroidism, adequate carbohydrate intake is needed to help prevent inadvertently decreasing the amount of thyroid hormones (T3 and T4) in the "free" and active form in the bloodstream. The Atkins Diet is too low in carbohydrate for most people with hypothyroidism can aggravate the problems of low thyroid function. On the other hand, too much carbohydrate intake can over stimulate the production of excess insulin and cause more fat to be stored instead of being burned for energy.

NATURAL PROGESTERONE – Dr. John Lee, a pioneer in natural progesterone research and treatment, says that if your T4 and T3 levels are normal and your TSH is high-normal or slightly higher than normal, natural progesterone may be all you need to balance your thyroid chemistry, especially if you are taking estrogen only or estrogen and progesterone. If you have any doubts about whether to take natural progesterone, have your progesterone level tested either via blood or saliva one week before your period is due to see if you are deficient. The dose of natural progesterone that works well for most women is one-quarter teaspoon of a 20mg transdermal cream, used once to twice per day, or about 20–40 mg/day, days 14 to 28 of the cycle. Post menopause, use daily for three weeks of every month.

THYROID EXTRACT – Thyroid extract is often superior to other forms of replacement thyroid hormone. At least part of the reason for this is that most synthetic forms of thyroid hormone only contain T4, whereas thyroid extract contains both T4 (thyroxine) and T3 (triiodothyronine). It is generally assumed that no one has any problem converting T4 to T3 in the thyroid and in other tissues of the body, but that is not always the case. Some people clearly benefit from supplemental T3. Physicians who see a lot of thyroid patients have recognised for years that occasionally patients simply do not feel as well taking pure thyroxine as they do when taking either desiccated thyroid or a compounded synthetic T4 and T3 formulation.

A recent study in The New England Journal of Medicine (Vol. 340, No. 8, pp.424-29, 469-70, Feb. 11, 1999) demonstrated that patients with hypothyroidism showed greater improvements in mood and neuropsychological functioning...if they received treatment with thyroid extract (Armour Thyroid, (T3, T4) rather than Thyroxine (T4). The authors also detected biochemical evidence that thyroid hormone action was greater... after treatment with thyroid extract - which is a desiccated form of thyroid hormone.

Numerous studies have examined the merits of replacing both T3 and T4 versus T4 alone. Some of these studies have been done in normal subjects; other studies have been carried out in patients with psychiatric illnesses, often depression. A common finding in several studies is that patients who are taking some form of T3 supplement feel better, in some subjective or objective measurements of mood or cognitive function, than those taking T4 alone. For example, see the overview of the study published in the 1999 study in the New England Journal of Medicine. (Vol. 340, Feb. 11, 1999)

An Endocrinology Clinic in Latvia did a T3/T4 Combination Study that was published in The New England Journal of Medicine in February 1999. These investigators asked the question: Do hypothyroid patients feel just as well taking pure T4 as they do when they are switched, without knowing it, to a combination of T4 + T3?

The authors studied 33 hypothyroid patients who were randomly assigned to take either their usual dose of T4 for 5 weeks or to take slightly less T4 plus a small dose of T3, so that the total amount of hormone, from a biological standpoint, was the same. After 5 weeks, the patients were switched to the other thyroid hormone regimen. The assignment to a particular regimen was done in random order: some people took T4 first and other people took T4 + T3 first. The study was also "blinded" so that neither the patients nor the doctors knew whether they were taking T4 or the T4 + T3 combination. The patients were given a battery of psychological tests as well as questionnaires that assessed their mood. The tests were given after 5 weeks of their usual T4 dose and after 5 weeks of the T4 + T3 combination.

Compared to T4 therapy, the T4 + T3 therapy was associated with a slight rise in the pulse rate, but no differences in blood pressure or serum cholesterol. Certain cognitive tests, like the ability to recall a series of numbers or draw a certain shape from memory were slightly better with the combination of T4 and T3. Perhaps more importantly, measures of mood, especially depression, low energy anger was improved with the combined regimen. When patients were asked whether they preferred the first treatment or the second treatment (not knowing which was the T4 and which was the T4 + T3), 20 preferred the T4 + T3 combination, 11 had no preference 2 preferred the T4 alone.

Treatment begins with small doses of thyroid hormone, because too large a dose can cause serious side effects. However, large doses may be necessary. The starting dose and the rate of increase are especially small in older people, who are often most at risk of side effects. The dose is gradually increased until the levels of thyroid-stimulating hormone in the person's blood return to normal. During pregnancy, doses may need to be adjusted.

If hypothyroidism is optimally treated so that TSH, free T3 and free T4 are in the desirable ranges, metabolism is generally improved to normal unless there are other hormone, medication, dietary, exercise or mineral deficiencies, etc.

For more information visit: www.redwoodnhrt.com.au or call 1300 304 638

Part 3

FOR THE WOMEN

If you've opened up a newspaper or turned on the television or even listened to the radio during the last several months, you've more than likely heard the debate on hormone replacement therapy, which we discussed earlier. If you're a woman and entering menopause, suffering PMS or hormone induced weight gain, you are no doubt very confused.

Women's hormonal fluctuations play havoc with their systems. This may vary widely within a single day and drive you and your family 'crazy'. A long-term decline in sex hormone levels produce symptoms such as dry skin, brittle hair, loss of libido, mood swings, hot flushes, night sweats, vaginal dryness and itching, ageing skin, increased chance of heart disease, osteoporosis, colon cancer and mental deterioration.

This usually begins around the age of 40; however, it can start by the early thirties and even as early as the twenties in some cases.

Hormone imbalance results in a variety of symptoms:

- Estrogen dominance
- Menopause
- Osteoporosis
- PMS
- Fertility
- Weight and hormones

ESTROGEN DOMINANCE

Estrogen, essential for living, but can cause mayhem for your body and the rest of your hormones if unbalanced!
Take this simple test to see if you may have a problem with estrogen dominance:

I feel anxious and irritable before a period	5	
I have polycystic ovary syndrome	20	
I am experiencing weight gain particularly in my hips and thighs	5	
I have breast cancer	5	
I have taken "the pill" for more than 6 months now or before in my life	5	
I suffer depression and sadness before my period	5	
I suffer frequently dry eyes	5	
I have endometriosis	10	
I feel fatigued and tired most of the time	5	
I have an autoimmune disorder	20	
I have fibrocystic breast disease	5	
I am infertile	10	
I suffer irregular menstrual cycles frequently	5	
I have fibroids	10	
I have terrible trouble sleeping prior to a period	5	
I have suffered a miscarriage in the first trimester	10	
I have been diagnosed with osteoporosis	10	
I suffer PMS	10	
I have low thyroid function	5	
I suffer water retention and bloating of the abdomen	5	
I have yellowish skin discoloration	5	
TOTAL		

See how you scored:

10-15 – Mild Estrogen Dominance
15-30 – Moderate Estrogen Dominance
30+   – Severe Estrogen Dominance

The result of too much estrogen relative to progesterone is estrogen dominance. It is the chief cause of PMS, fibroids, endometriosis, polycystic ovary syndrome, infertility and other hormonal imbalances. Under the influence of too much estrogen women feel bloated, irritable, fatigued and have sugar cravings.

As we know estrogen, even our own milder estrogen, is a very powerful hormone. It has the potential to lower metabolism by suppressing thyroid function and by storing blood sugar as fat. Estrogen also stimulates the growth of breast and uterus tissue.

XENO-ESTROGENS (HIDDEN ESTROGENS)

There has also been much recent research done on a syndrome called estrogen dominance. This occurs when estrogen and progesterone are out of balance caused by too much estrogen and not enough progesterone. This imbalance is exacerbated by the massive amounts of xenobiotics present in the environment.

Xenobiotics are created primarily from industrial chemicals, animal growth hormones, by plastic products that have entered our food chain, through pesticides and herbicide application.

These xenobiotics are causing havoc with women's (and men's) balance of estrogen and progesterone. In women as young as 14 or 15 years old it can create many short and long term health problems from PMS, abdominal cramps, water retention through to infertility.

To protect against estrogen dominance the ratio of progesterone to estradiol in women should be 200:1. Normal progesterone levels for postmenopausal women is less than 100picog/ml, for menstruating women during days 19-22 of their cycle 200-500picog/ml.

HELP! I'M UNBALANCED!

All of these estrogenic effects are supposed to be balanced by progesterone, but in most women, they are not. It is important that estrogen dominance is addressed as a matter of priority as it can influence all your other hormones. Here are some steps to mastering the estrogen-balancing act.

MINIMISE EXPOSURE TO XENO-ESTROGENS

- Avoid pollution, pesticides, solvents plastics as much as possible.
- Avoid synthetic HRT and the contraceptive pill
- Improve liver functioning by avoiding excessive alcohol consumption and high-processed food.
- Exercise regularly

MAKE PROGESTERONE WORK FOR YOU

Natural progesterone will help to protect your breasts and uterus from the cancer-promoting effects of estrogen.

Natural progesterone will increase metabolism, burn fat, relieve depression and anxiety, act as a natural diuretic, normalise blood clotting, stimulate new bone formation and stabilise blood sugar. Successful ovulation is required for the ovary to produce adequate progesterone.

If you are suffering PMS, hot flushes, going through menopause or concerned about osteoporosis, estrogen may be the key culprit and supplementation of progesterone could be well advised. To determine whether you are in fact suffering estrogen dominance you will need to have a saliva test and consult with your physician.

Should you be estrogen dominant then progesterone applied transdermally, once or twice per day, may be exactly what you need.

For more information visit: www.redwoodnhrt.com.au

or call 1300 304 638

MENOPAUSE

For at least thirty years many doctors and scientists have raised safety questions about conventional practices in treating women with hormones, especially estrogens derived from horse urine. For at least a decade we have had strong scientific evidence that there are many women who have gotten serious illnesses from the most commonly used of these synthetic hormone medications, Premarin and Prempro. For several decades many doctors, pharmacists and other practitioners, as well as women with this concern, have sought to understand this topic and offer better solutions. Following the WHI findings you may have stopped your HRT, as millions of menopausal women worldwide did are now suffering the consequences. This information will provide you with some relief.

THE CHANGE OF LIFE

Menopause changes your life. You will never be the same again!
As you enter menopause, your ovaries stop producing estrogen and progesterone. As a result, your menstrual cycle will start to change and you will eventually reach a point when you stop having your period. This is a perfectly normal change that all women go through, usually between the ages of 45 and 55, with the average being 51, although it can occur much earlier in some cases.

ALL TOO FAMILIAR

During menopause, your body goes through a series of changes as it readjusts to the loss of estrogen and progesterone caused by the onset of menopause. During this readjustment period, known as peri-menopause, women can experience a wide range of symptoms including:

- Hot flushes
- Depression
- Irregular menstrual cycle
- Night sweats
- Increasing vaginal dryness, itching and discomfort
- Palpitations or bouts of rapid heartbeat
- Mood swings and generally unstable or erratic behavior.

- Breast tenderness.
- Painful sexual intercourse.
- Loss of libido and sexual desire
- Sleep disturbances
- Emotional instability
- Urinary frequency and frequent yeast infections
- Weight gain
- Bone loss
- Low energy and fatigue
- Bleeding gums
- Body odour
- Brittle fingernails
- Breast tenderness
- Burning tongue
- Memory lapses
- Sore joints and muscles
- Clammy feeling
- Tingling in the extremities
- Dizziness and light-headedness
- Fatigue
- Feelings of anxiety, dread and apprehension
- Hair loss or thinning
- Headaches
- Increase in facial hair
- Indigestion and nausea
- Itchy, crawly skin

Again, these changes are perfectly natural and are a normal part of menopause, but vary in degree from woman to woman. For some women the onset of menopause is horror, for others it is a breeze.

MENOPAUSE WITH A DIFFERENCE

The symptoms of menopause, when they occur and how long they last, are just as individual as the menstrual cycle itself. Women can find as many similarities in their experiences as they can find problems specific to themselves. One of those shared experiences is that natural menopause is a gradual process. The body has years to adjust to it.

This is important, because the transition process - with the integrity of the ovaries remaining intact and producing hormones - marks the great difference between a natural menopause and a sudden menopause.

A NATURAL MENOPAUSE

Natural menopause is a process. It begins quietly with a few peri-menopause symptoms but can become quite loud at its menopause peak. Eventually, the body calms down again in post menopause.

The term peri-menopause often is used to refer to the year or few years preceding menopause, when a woman may begin experiencing erratic periods and changes as just described. Some women do not experience these worrying changes until menopause actually occurs.

Approximately 2 to 4 years before the last period, ovulation becomes irregular and eventually ceases. The ovaries continue to produce some estrogen, but progesterone production is dependent on ovulation. Therefore, estrogen builds up the lining of the uterus, but if ovulation does not occur, progesterone is not present to cause the uterine lining to slough off on a regular basis. Instead, a woman bleeds erratically as the endometrium breaks away uncleanly, due to the months of build up. This can lead to irregular cycles-light flow, heavy flow, skipped periods, or more or less frequent periods.

When menopause does occur, it is marked by the end of your period. Other changes that occur include the completion of the fertile years, a decline in levels of estrogen, testosterone and the termination of progesterone production from the ovaries.

After menopause the ovaries no longer produce hormones at their previous levels. Although estrogen is typically only produced at 40% of previous produced amounts it is still adequate for most women. It is NOT only a lack of estrogen that creates the problems. It is the lack of progesterone. If a woman's body is given back the progesterone it can no longer produce, menopausal symptoms will diminish significantly and disappear in most women.

A PREMATURE MENOPAUSE

Sudden menopause can result from a variety of conditions that instantly render a woman's ovaries incapable of producing the crucial female hormones estrogen and progesterone, as well as the male hormone testosterone. This immediate depletion throws the woman's body into a hormonal tailspin. Sudden menopause can be induced by surgical intervention (hysterectomy) or by ovarian damage. Ovarian damage can be a result of anorexia nervosa, chemotherapy, radiation treatment and even certain conventional medications.

Whether sudden menopause follows surgery or ovarian damage, the body may react to the resulting drastic hormonal changes by manifesting such symptoms as hot flushes, night sweats, vaginal dryness, decreased libido, memory loss and mood changes.

MENOPAUSE FACTS MOST DOCTORS WON'T TELL YOU

Menopause can be a smooth journey for some women and a rocky road for others. For all there are choices. There are other methods of treatment. For e.g. naturally derived, bio-identical hormones. They are safe and they offer a wealth of benefits including:

- Prevention of osteoporosis and restoration of bone strength
- Reduced hot flushes and reduced vaginal dryness/thinning
- Better maintenance of muscle mass and strength
- Protection against heart disease and stroke as natural progesterone acts like a natural diuretic
- Improved cholesterol levels plus natural progesterone's promotion of thermogenesis
- Reduced risk of endometrial cancer and breast cancer
- Reduced risk of depression
- Improved sleep and better mood, concentration and memory
- Prevention of senility and Alzheimer's disease
- Improved libido

> **CHANGING SAFELY**
>
> "The advantages of NHRT for menopausal and peri-menopausal women are now quite clear. They include all the well known benefits of HRT and more, *with very few of the unwanted effects and risks associated with the man-made variety.*" [Ibid, p.31]

"AM I LOSING MY MIND? WHAT IS GOING ON?"

In addition to the biological factors in menopause that you may face, there can be challenges in your relationships, jobs or other life issues that you felt quite capable of handling before menopause. Your hormones can dramatically affect your mood, energy, vitality and sexuality. If you do not successfully treat the hormonal issues of menopause, you may have more difficulty resolving the other issues in your life.

With unbalanced and insufficient hormones you could be operating out of tiredness rather than vitality, sleep de-privation rather than being rested, mood swings rather than emotional stability even disease rather than health. The stress from unresolved issues of life can result in significant glandular fatigue then further hormonal reduction and imbalance.

MY LIBIDO IS IN LIMBO!

One of the biggest complaints of women approaching menopause is that they have no sex drive. Funny enough, it is the husband's complaint about his wife's menopause aswell! That coupled with his complaint of not enough blankets on the bed in winter and waking up wet from your sweat!

When the ovaries shut down during menopause, the quantity of testosterone produced is cut in half. Women who are taking natural estrogen and progesterone to combat menopause usually regain some of this loss of sex drive, however, a small number of women do not. Some researchers believe that these women may be more sensitive to the accompanying loss of testosterone.

Davis (1998) points out that using androgens with

postmenopausal women successfully increases their sexual desire. However, the bigger picture is that androgen (testosterone) levels fall significantly throughout the reproductive years and probably affect desire from an early age (Longcope 1998; Gelfand 1999). Circulating levels of androgens play an important role in psychological and sexual changes that occur in menopause, whether naturally or surgically induced.

Over the past decade Dr John Moran of the Optimal Health Clinic in London has pioneered hormone replacement therapy, prescribing testosterone to women. He has noticed that many women respond positively when a small amount of testosterone is added to their natural hormone replacement program. Libido seems to be restored.

Results from clinical studies showed that in some women a combination of estrogen and testosterone replacement provided greater improvement in psychological (e.g., fatigue, lack of concentration depression) and sexual function (e.g., inability to have an orgasm and decreased libido) than estrogen alone (Bachmann 1999, 2001; Gelfand 1999; Sarrel 1999)

BUT MUM DID IT WITH NO HELP AT ALL

Environment, responsibilities, foods and products have changed a lot since your mum went through menopause. So don't be afraid to ask for help! Menopause can be a challenge and it is important to get it right to ensure you can stay sane and enjoy life! If you have heard uncomfortable stories from your friends or on the news, know that you can do it all differently.

DIET – Eat organic, whole, non-processed food as much as possible. Enjoy a low fat, high fibre diet. Eat essential fatty acids to help to maintain healthy hormonal receptor sites. Omega-3 and omega-6 essential fatty acids from cold water fish (tuna) and healthy oils (flaxseed oil or perilla oil). Limit intake of alcohol and avoid smoking.

VITAMINS AND MINERALS – Take a comprehensive vitamin

and mineral supplement. This list is of optimal levels for menopause.

- Vitamin C: Take 2.5 – 6 grams daily
- Vitamin D3: Take 400 – 1500 IU daily.
- Vitamin B complex – including B6, B12 and folic acid.
- Take 1000 mg calcium daily and 400 mg of magnesium in a combined dose to prevent bone loss.
- Vitamin E: Take 400 IU daily can help raise progesterone levels.
- CoQ10: Take 100-300 mg daily (those over 40).

Other botanical nutrients that can help ease menopausal systems are: black cohosh, dong quai, motherwort, liquorice root and red raspberry.

INDOLE 3 CARBINOL – Take 150mg – 300mg of I3C daily for the beneficial effects it has on estrogens.

EXERCISE – More aerobic and weight-bearing exercise is important for menopause, not to mention for healthy bones.

NHRT – Natural hormone replacement treatment by carefully selected bio-identical hormones. Estrogen, progesterone, testosterone and DHEA are all commonly prescribed and most often in the form of cream or troche.

The optimal approach to managing your menopause is for you to have a significant understanding of how your own body works, uncovering and reducing possible personal risk factors related to female organ disease and making choices for treatment accordingly. It is also crucial, if you choose treatment using natural hormones, that you use the best quality combinations and doses of bio-identical hormones.

A HEALTHY PRESCRIPTION FOR THE CHANGE

ESTROGEN – We have established that estrogen plays a vital role in your body. The need to modulate the relative levels of the primary female hormones is of critical importance throughout life. Proper hormone replacement therapy not only alleviates menopausal symptoms but also helps prevent common disorders, such as PMS, endometriosis, several types of cancer, sexual dysfunction, fibroid tumors, osteoporosis and possibly alzheimer's disease. Many diseases are linked to either excessive or deficient estrogen levels, particularly compared to the amount of progesterone available.

Despite all the problems estrogen can cause when in excess, in a balanced amount it can actually prevent some of the long-term health risks. By taking natural estrogen replacement you can restore the estrogen levels that you had prior to menopause. Don't forget estrogen does:

- Enhance skin smoothness, firmness and elasticity (Castelo-Branco et al. 1998)
- Enhance moistness of skin and mucous membranes
- Enhance muscle tone
- Reduce genital atrophy and enhanced sex drive (Head 1998)
- Reduce menopausal miseries such as hot flushes and anxiety (Vincent 2000)
- Reduce risk of heart disease and osteoporosis (Kaufert et al. 1998; Sites 1998)
- Reduce risk of colon cancer
- Improve memory and neurological function (Sherwin 1994; Jacobs et al. 1998)
- Provide protection from alzheimer's disease (Resnick et al. 1997; DeGregorio et al. 1998)
- Enhance immune function
- Improve feeling of well-being

The benefits of estrogen make it desirable for most menopausal women to maintain youthful levels of this hormone. The question is: Do you want estrogen without increasing your risk of cancer? Therefore, if you require estrogen supplementation then you should consider the natural combinations Triest, Biest or Estriol alone. (Refer to estrogen section of this book).

PROGESTERONE – Progesterone is important during the menstruation years and as beneficial during the menopausal years. Levels of progesterone actually decline faster than estrogen levels in the peri-menopausal years, which results in hot flushes, night sweats, irregular periods, mood changes, vaginal dryness and discomfort. For this reason, progesterone is often preferred over estrogen as the initial hormone replacement treatment for menopausal symptoms. Rather than regulate the menstrual cycle of a menopausal woman, natural progesterone helps with many of the symptoms of menopause. Progesterone also balances the effects of estrogen and should always be taken in conjunction with estrogen therapy even after hysterectomy.

TESTOSTERONE – Testosterone needs to be introduced only once you have balanced your estrogen and progesterone. Caution also needs to be employed if you are taking DHEA or pregnenolone as these hormones convert to testosterone. In women, excess testosterone can have undesired side effects, such as acne, baldness, enlarged clitoris, increased facial or chest hair and deepening of the voice. Side effects to low conservative dosages are very rare.

For more information visit: www.redwoodnhrt.com.au
or call 1300 304 638

OSTEOPOROSIS

You have a higher chance of getting osteoporosis if:

- You reached menopause before age 48
- You have had surgery to remove ovaries before menopause
- You are not getting enough calcium
- You do not exercise enough
- You are deficient in Vitamin D
- You are a smoker
- You have a history of osteoporosis in your family
- You consume excessive amounts of alcohol
- You have a thin body and small bone frame
- You have fair skin (Caucasian or Asian race)
- You have hyperthyroidism
- You use oral steroids long-term

Osteoporosis is a condition in which the bones become porous and liable to fracture.

Bones are just like all parts of our bodies, they consist of living tissue that breaks down and is constantly renewed. Estrogen and progesterone are essential to this process of renewal. Hormone levels, therefore, directly relate to bone renewal or lack there of.

HOW TO MAKE HEALTHY BONES

Bone metabolism is a complex process in which production and deterioration work along side one another. Each of our bodies 206 bones harbour cells that continually deposit a protein framework made from collagen. Minerals from the blood then attach to this matrix and harden into bone. Those same bones also contain cells that can break down that structure. As we grow the osteoblasts, the cells that make bone, tend to dominate. However, later in life, with the influence of a variety of conditions such as depression, steroid use and mineral and hormone deficiencies allow the osteoclasts, the cells that break down bone, to take over (Northrup 2001: 372). It is the latter that can have the most predominant effect. However natural progesterone and estrogen supplementation regenerate the osteoblasts, encouraging bone growth, preventing and reversing the effects of osteoporosis.

MILK IS NOT ENOUGH

The most common myth about osteoporosis is that insufficient calcium intake is the culprit. Indeed in countries where we find the highest consumption of dairy food we find a corresponding correlation of the highest rates of osteoporosis. This is more of a problem of poor absorption and utilisation of available calcium and the lack of other essential minerals, which contributes to the bone density loss.

Other factors also known to damage bone-building cells include smoking and drinking excess alcohol, as well as eating disorders such as bulimia and anorexia, excess aerobic activity and athletics can cause amenorrhea (lack of menstruation). This type of estrogen deficiency causes the bones to weaken prematurely. This gradual change in the bones is not painful until a fracture or break occurs, therefore, osteoporosis goes unrecognised and it is commonly known as the "silent disease" (Buckman 1999:13-15).

THE TRUTH ABOUT YOUR BONES

Contrary to popular belief bone density loss is long underway before menopause, at least 5 to 20 years in fact, when the ovaries are still functioning and estrogen levels are high.

The ratio of progesterone to estrogen has a greater impact on your bones and osteoporosis. While estrogen is proven to slow bone loss, progesterone is proven to cause bone re-growth.

Dr John Lee is known for his work showing women how to restore bone tissue. In a study over ten years with 63 women, he showed that natural progesterone replacement has the capacity, to restore bone loss. He found that a natural progesterone cream resulted in a remarkable increase in bone mineral density, in some patients by 20% to 25% in the first year. Age was not an obstacle to bone restoration. Similar studies using synthetic hormone replacement, progestins, have only hinted at a small bone-building benefit (3-5%) (Wright & Morgenthaler 1997:66).

None of these synthetic progestin replacement studies have established the positive affects that have been firmly reinforced by the use of natural progesterone replacement.

BUILD BONES NATURALLY

- Eat plenty of green vegetables, whole grains and fibre
- Regular weight bearing exercise
- Reduce your stress
- Reduce tea & coffee consumption, excessive alcohol and smoking
- Magnesium 400 – 600mg daily
- Vitamin C 200mg daily
- Zinc 15 – 30mg daily
- Vitamin B6 50mg daily
- Calcium 800 – 1000mg daily
- Beta-carotene 15mg daily
- Vitamin D – get a good dose of fresh air and sunlight will aid absorption of calcium
- Natural progesterone cream 15 – 30mg daily

Estrogen, while having a "bone benefit," is only truly effective for approximately five years after menopause. While natural estrogen replacement slows bone loss, it ignores bone re-building. Progesterone may be more important than estrogen for preventing and treating osteoporosis because progesterone is directly involved in the production of bone-forming cells called osteoblasts. This is why natural progesterone replacement is combined with natural estrogen to assist in reversing the effects of osteoporosis.

Many women use a transdermal natural progesterone cream to provide for direct absorption of progesterone into the bloodstream. Natural progesterone treatment in the form of a cream or troche will provide optimum protection against osteoporosis. (15-30mg daily)

In addition to progesterone, supplementation with at least 800 – 1000mg a day of calcium along with magnesium, zinc, beta-carotene, vitamin D and vitamin K are essential in the prevention of osteoporosis.

ARE MY BONES SICK?

The best way to find out whether you have osteoporosis is by having a bone density test. Many women have started to lose bone after age 30 so it's a good idea to have a bone density test quite young, maybe 35, to have a base level to compare with later on.

The most sophisticated method for diagnosing osteoporosis is a DEXA (dual energy x-rays absorptiometry) scanning test. A bone mineral density test measures the mineral density in the bone by bouncing a dual photon beam of light off the bone, measuring the difference in the density between bone and soft tissue. This shows how porous the bones have become and at what risk you are of having a fracture or degree of osteoporosis.

The bone density test can only diagnose whether or not you have osteoporosis. The next step is to find out the cause of osteoporosis. In most postmenopausal women, it is estrogen deficiency.

For more information visit: <u>www.redwoodnhrt.com.au</u>
or call 1300 304 638

PREMENSTRUAL SYNDROME

Premenstrual syndrome, or PMS, is a range of symptoms that can cause annoying physical and/or behavioral changes in the week or two prior to menstruation. The most marked changes usually occur the week before the onset of menstruation, but milder symptoms may occur at the time of ovulation (14 days before the onset of menstruation) and become progressively worse. The symptoms should stop either at the beginning of menstruation, or at least, by the end of menstruation.

The relative deficiency of progesterone to estrogen in the second half of the menstrual cycle (the luteal phase) may be the cause of PMS symptoms, especially the emotionally related ones.

THAT CRAZY TIME OF THE MONTH

PMS differs from all other hormone related disorders because the diagnosis does not depend on the type of symptoms you suffer from, but on the time when your symptoms appear and disappear.

Dr. Katharina Dalton of the U.K., a leading specialist who first used the term "premenstrual syndrome", defines it as "the presence of recurrent symptoms before menstruation with the complete absence of symptoms after menstruation". Doctors have identified at least 150 symptoms that occur in PMS but fortunately, because all of us are different, no one has all of them!

Dr. Katharina Dalton knew this back in the late 50s when she pioneered the use of natural progesterone to balance estrogen in PMS patients with great success. Over the years she and physicians like Dr. John Lee, have treated thousands of women worldwide in this way. The great majority of patients report remarkable improvement in their PMS symptoms including the elimination of premenstrual water retention, cramping, tearfulness and weight gain.

I DON'T USUALLY ACT LIKE THIS!

- Increased anger and loss of control
- Sudden unexplained mood swings
- Extra emotional over-responsiveness
- Unexplained crying and sadness
- Anxious and irritable
- Decreased concentration
- Confused and forgetful
- Depression and possibly suicidal thoughts
- Nightmares
- Bloating – fluid retention
- Breast tenderness
- Weight gain
- Acne and skin outbreaks
- Dizziness
- Migraine headaches
- Joint aches, muscle pain and backaches
- Reduced sex drive
- Uncontrollable food cravings
- Constipation or diarrhea
- Sweating, shakiness or even seizures

HELP! WHAT CAN I DO?

Hormones and lifestyle influence the severity of PMS. Here are a few ideas to help keep you sane during the onset of that dreaded time of the month.

EXERCISE REGULARLY – Exercise at least 3 times per week.

EAT WELL – Limit your salt intake to 3 grams or less per day and avoid caffeine, foods high in refined white flour and sugar products. Minimise your intake of processed foods, alcohol, chocolate, fatty foods and nicotine. Cut your red meat consumption to once or twice a week only and increase your fluid intake.

NUTRITIONAL SUPPLEMENTS – VITAMINS AND MINERALS.

- VITAMIN B6 - It is best taken with the other B vitamins (B1, B2, B12) in the form of a "B-Complex". Supplementation of Vitamin B6 should not exceed 100mg a day.
- VITAMIN E – Vitamin E may be helpful taken in doses from 150 to 300mg a day.
- MAGNESIUM – Best taken in oral doses from 300 to 500mg a day. Magnesium may relieve premenstrual mood changes. Magnesium supplementation should not be taken at the same time of day as calcium supplement.
- EVENING PRIMROSE OIL – Taking 3 – 4 grams daily with meals may assist in correcting abnormal fatty acid metabolism and may bring relief of PMS symptoms.

NATURAL PROGESTERONE CREAM

WHY SUFFER? MANAGE YOUR PMS.

To understand how progesterone will help you, you need to understand how it works.

Estrogen is the dominant sex hormone the first week after menstruation. During the final two weeks after ovulation progesterone levels rise to take over the dominance. If this balance is out and either too much estrogen is produced, or too little progesterone is secreted, problems arise. If this occurs it allows an abnormal dominance of estrogen resulting in low progesterone side effects e.g. water retention, weight gain, mood swings etc.

Step one, in considering natural progesterone treatment, is to establish a full hormonal medical background. It is helpful to keep a menstrual chart for 2 – 3 months prior to treatment. This chart is most important to record the timing of symptoms, thus, the exact dates of symptoms and menstruation are essential.

The amount of the progesterone you may need is very individual and requires saliva tests and/or blood tests at specific periods of the menstrual cycle. This testing can determine if your PMS is associated with estrogen dominance (lack of progesterone). A low progesterone/estradiol ratio on your test report indicates estrogen dominance and the likelihood of PMS. Follow up tests once you have begun treatment, usually every 3 – 6 months, helps you and your doctor assess the dose and amend it if needed.

From the symptom information and the saliva and/or blood assessment your doctor can make an educated decision as to the dosage of your progesterone. Individually customised medication makes this possible. The dosage of progesterone varies depending on the individual needs. Progesterone can be prescribed by your doctor to be taken continuously or cyclically throughout the menstrual cycle.

EXAMPLE OF PROGESTERONE THERAPY CYCLE:

Day 1 – 14 NO PROGESTERONE THERAPY

Day 14 – 21 PROGESTERONE (generally between 50 – 200mg twice daily)

Day 21 – 28 PROGESTERONE (generally between 100 – 400mg twice daily)

INTO THE BLOODSTREAM THROUGH THE SKIN

Natural progesterone cream is the best option in the management of your PMS. The natural progesterone is absorbed through the skin directly into the bloodstream bypassing the liver so that the maximum amount of progesterone is absorbed and can be used in the body. The cream is best absorbed when applied to the skin on the inner forearm, but can also be applied to the skin on the stomach or thighs, once or twice per day.

LIKE APPLES AND ORANGES

"Wild yam cream" available in health food stores is NOT natural progesterone. They are apples and oranges! These wild yam creams often contain little or no progesterone at all and are often an expensive and ineffective treatment. Some of these products advertise that they are derived from wild yams or contain wild yam extract. Other products use terms like "balancing formula" and "precursor to the hormone progesterone" in their product descriptions. Some even imply that they contain natural progesterone. Wild yam DOES NOT contain progesterone and your body doesn't convert wild yam extract into progesterone. Micronised progesterone, the real pharmaceutical grade natural progesterone, is a prescription only medication, available through a compounding pharmacy ONLY. Don't waste your time, energy, money or health on these products or you will be bitterly disappointed.

For more information visit: www.redwoodnhrt.com.au
or call 1300 304 638

FERTILITY

Natural progesterone:

- Makes the survival of the fertilised egg possible
- Maintains the uterus lining, which feeds the ovum & resultant embryo
- Surges when a woman ovulates and is a source of libido
- Is essential to prevent miscarriage. A significant drop in progesterone levels or blockade of progesterone receptor sites during the first 10 – 12 weeks of pregnancy may result in the loss of the embryo (miscarriage).

THE MONTHLY INFLUENCE

The proper amount of natural progesterone is crucial to a woman who is trying to become pregnant. Natural progesterone prepares the uterine wall for implantation of the fertilised egg. Without adequate progesterone, the egg will be expelled. Natural progesterone treatment can also be used to induce fertility when there appears to be dysfunction with ovulation.

Interestingly, the word progesterone is given its name because of its vital supportive role in gestation (Latin: gestare), a fact that sheds some insight into its importance in the reproductive process.

Modern science confirms that progesterone is the most essential hormone for conception and for the survival of the fertilised egg and the foetus throughout gestation.

At ovulation, progesterone levels rise rapidly from 2 – 3 mg/day to an average of 22 – 25 mg/per day, peaking as high as 30 mg/day. If fertilisation does not occur in ten or twelve days, progesterone levels fall dramatically, triggering the shedding of the uterus (the menstrual cycle).

In the instance when pregnancy does occur, however, progesterone production is taken over by the placenta which secretes an ever increasing supply reaching 300 – 400 mg/day during the third trimester! A lot of progesterone!

MAKING A BABY? NEED PROGESTERONE.

Research indicates that natural progesterone can raise the progesterone levels in women to help them conceive and carry pregnancy to full term.

Before you begin the expensive and often unsuccessful process of working with a fertility clinic, I strongly recommend that you read Dr. Lee's book, "What Your Doctor May Not Tell You About Menopause", which will give you a detailed look at how your hormones work.

Progesterone influences the inability to conceive a baby. This can be caused by inadequate production during the luteal phase of the cycle.

Dr. Lee had a number of patients in his practice that had been unable to conceive. For two to four months he had them use natural progesterone from days 5 to 26 in the cycle (stopping on day 26 to bring on menstruation). Using the progesterone prior to ovulation effectively suppressed ovulation. After a few months of this, he had them stop progesterone use. If you still have follicles left, they seem to respond to a few months of progesterone suppression with enthusiasm. This resulted in the successful maturation and release of an egg. His patients, some of whom had been trying to get pregnant for years, had very good results trying to conceive with this method.

STAYING PREGNANT

Progesterone also influences the ability to carry a baby to term.

Progesterone is essential to prevent the premature shedding of the supportive lining of the uterus, a significant drop in progesterone levels or blockade of progesterone receptor sites during the first 10 – 12 weeks of pregnancy may result in the loss of the embryo (miscarriage). Women with a history of miscarriage should begin using progesterone cream as soon as they know they have ovulated, to supplement their own progesterone and offset any environmental estrogen effects. (Using progesterone before ovulation can create a hormonal signal that tells the brain not to ovulate).

THE PITTER-PATTER OF TINY FEET

If you are pregnant, keep using the progesterone every day in normal doses. Its fine to use it throughout your pregnancy and it's important not to stop it until your third trimester when the placenta is making sufficient progeterone that it won't notice if there's a drop of 15 to 30 mg a day.

Research by the British hormone researcher Katherina Dalton, M.D., indicates that babies born to mothers who used natural progesterone during pregnancy are normal and in fact, are larger, calmer and smarter. She reported that women who use a properly formulated compounded progesterone cream during the first 19 – 20 weeks of pregnancy produce healthier, more intelligent children. Also in her 1968 study she found that none of the women receiving antenatal progesterone experienced toxemia during the pregnancy.

Used from conception to delivery, applied primarily to abdomen, breasts, low back and upper thighs, progesterone tends to prevent the skin from stretching. The cream is also useful for post partum depression, which many women experience after childbirth.

If you find out that you are not pregnant, stop taking the progesterone on day 28 of your cycle or whenever the last day of your cycle normally occurs.

THE RIGHT AMOUNT FOR A SMART BABY

Progesterone can also be compounded into various dosage forms such as: cream, gel, vaginal pessaries and troches. The dose of progesterone is dependent upon an individual woman's needs and the specific dosage form of progesterone that is chosen.

In order to mimic a regular menstrual cycle, therapy with progesterone is usually started a few days after ovulation and is continued until either menses occurs or pregnancy is confirmed. If pregnancy is achieved, treatment with progesterone may be continued for up to 10 to 12 weeks. By this time, the placenta (the organ in the womb that nourishes the foetus) is producing sufficient amounts of progesterone for the remainder of the pregnancy.

For more information visit: www.redwoodnhrt.com.au
or call 1300 304 638

WEIGHT AND HORMONES

Women have to struggle three times as hard to lose half the weight a man does. Hormone imbalances cause weight gain and can actually be made worse by the wrong type of food choices.

According to Dr Marcus Laux, an internationally renowned naturopathic physician and pre-eminent pioneer in the field of integrative medicine, obesity is a major risk factor in diabetes. Both obesity and diabetes are risk factors for the development of cardiovascular disease. It also increases the risk of developing high blood pressure, certain types of cancer, gout and gallbladder disease, compared to people of normal weight. It can also be related to problems such as sleep apnea (interrupted breathing during sleep), infertility in women and osteoarthritis.

TOP 5 REASONS WHY YOU DO NOT LOSE WEIGHT

SYNTHETIC HRT OR BIRTH CONTROL PILL

Synthetic estrogens and progestins used in conventional HRT and "the pill" cause weight gain. Not only do they make women gain weight they foil any attempts to lose weight. This weight gain is typical of the weight gain experienced in estrogen dominance.

UNDERACTIVE THYROID

Low thyroid function will cause weight gain. Estrogen dominance also inhibits thyroid function hence the weight piles on.

UNHEALTHY LIVER

The liver – the powerhouse of the body producing enzymes, balancing sugar levels and converting fat into energy! An unhealthy liver means your metabolism will be slowed and your weight will balloon. If the liver is not working properly, it will perpetuate the estrogen excess cycle by allowing estrogen to build up. In order to keep your liver functioning and fat burning you need to address your diet and make sure your vitamin and mineral intake is adequate.

LACK OF EXERCISE

No need to grab a leotard and hit the gym, but you do need to at least walk and do some weight bearing exercise. You've heard it before, but once again, inactivity will make you fat!

STRESS/DEPRESSION

Not having the time, energy or inclination to look after yourself, will cause weight gain. If you use food to control emotions, watch out for the weight. In fact, emotional eating may account for up to 75% of overeating.

When you are stressed your body produces excess amounts of cortisol. This helps you cope but it also destabilises your blood sugar levels and will cause you to gain weight. According to Dr Pamela Peeke, assistant clinical professor at the University of Maryland School of Medicine and author of 'Fight Fat After Forty,' comfort eating during stressful moments – which tend to be many – is one of the main reasons our waistlines expand.

NOT ESTROGEN AGAIN!

This time estrogen is putting on the kilos and causing problems with insulin and thyroid!

Estrogen is manufactured and stored in body fat, which closely links this hormone with weight gain. Women with estrogen dominance convert more food energy into fat instead of burning it as metabolic energy. They also tend to retain fluid and salt and to crave carbohydrates, which can lead to blood sugar problems and insulin imbalances. Synthetic HRT and "the pill" will increase your estrogen and fat will stay.

Excess estrogen can interfere with the function of thyroid and the action of thyroid hormones. This interference, causing fatigue, loss of energy a drop in metabolism can contribute to weight gain. Estrogen and thyroid hormones have opposing actions. Estrogen causes calories to be stored as fat, where as the thyroid hormones cause fat calories to be turned into usable energy.

Dr Lee suggests that estrogen inhibits thyroid actions in the cells, probably interfering with the binding of thyroid to its receptor. 'Estrogen competes with the thyroid hormone at the site of its receptor. In doing so, the thyroid hormone doesn't complete its purpose creating hypothyroid symptoms, despite normal serum levels of thyroid hormone'.

FIGHT THE BULGE WITH NHRT

The key to weight loss is hormonal health. All hormones must work together to achieve harmony in the body. So don't waste your time and money with diet and exercise if your hormones are out of kilter!

PROGESTERONE – You can use natural progesterone, an effective weight loss agent!

When progesterone is in short supply, women become "estrogen dominant," a condition that world health expert John R Lee MD describes as 'toxic to the body'. Estrogen dominance can cause damage to the pituitary gland and put stress on the liver function. The liver is required to process estrogen and to convert thyroid hormone to its active form.

Progesterone increases the sensitivity of estrogen receptors for estrogen and at a proper level inhibits the estrogen side effects. Symptoms of hypothyroidism occurring in patients, who are progesterone deficient, become less so when progesterone is added and a hormonal balance is attained.

DHEA & 7 KETO DHEA – Studies have shown DHEA to encourage weight loss and work against obesity. DHEA is said to raise the metabolism and decrease appetite and fat storage.

"DHEA is a very effective anti-obesity agent." claimed Dr Arthur Schwartsz, Vice President for Research and Programs in the Human Sciences at Temple University. He claims DHEA, may be the potential weapon against the battle of the bulge.

A study at Temple's University school of Medicine found that DHEA caused weight loss without a change in appetite. Recent research has begun to show how DHEA exerts its extraordinary weight loss effects.

Weight loss occurred because calories where converted to heat rather than fat claims Dr Schwartz. DHEA behaves similarly to thyroid hormone, by enhancing the metabolism.

In one study, extremely high doses of DHEA (1600mg per day) given for four weeks, caused a 31% decrease in body fat in four of five subjects with no overall weight change, implying a substantial increase in muscle mass. Their LDL levels also fell by 7.5% showing that DHEA may protect against cardiovascular disease as well.

Various studies have shown low levels of DHEA to be associated with obesity. A 1964 study found that DHEA was completely absent from urine samples of 32 elderly, obese diabetics. Obese people were also found to excrete less DHEA then people of normal weight. [Klatz & Goldman, Stopping the Clock: 69]

The ability of 7 KETO DHEA, a substance related to DHEA, to promote weight loss in overweight people has been investigated in one double-blind trial, which is a giant step for NHRT. Each person was given either a placebo or 100 mg of 7 KETO DHEA twice daily. After eight weeks, those receiving 7 KETO DHEA had lost more weight (6.34 pounds) and lowered their percentage of body fat (1.8%) further compared to those taking a placebo.

For more information visit: www.redwoodnhrt.com.au
or call 1300 304 638

FOR THE MEN

Men have hormones too! They experience hormonal deficiencies and fluctuations as women do!

As men age past 40, hormonal changes occur that inhibit physical, sexual and cognitive function. The outward appearance of a typical middle-aged male shows increased abdominal fat and shrinkage of muscle mass, a hallmark effect of hormone imbalance. Loss of a feeling of well-being, sometimes manifesting as depression, is a common complication of hormone imbalance in the ageing male. Until recently, these changes were attributed to "growing old," and men simply accepted it.

A remarkable amount of data has been compiled indicating that many of the diseases that middle-aged men begin experiencing, including depression, fatigue, abdominal weight gain, alterations in mood and cognition, decreased libido, erectile dysfunction, prostate disease and heart disease are directly related to hormone imbalances that are correctable with diet, exercise and natural hormones.

ANDROPAUSE – THE MALE MENOPAUSE

Andropause! Sometimes referred to as 'Male Menopause,' is a term that is becoming increasingly accepted. It may have a mythic status due to many men's "don't ask – don't tell" unwillingness to acknowledge the condition, yet, it is no joke!

Andropause refers to the gradual, but significant decline in testosterone, DHEA and growth hormone. There is a slow and relentless decline of testicular function and hence testosterone production.

Between the ages of 40 and 55, men can experience a condition similar to menopause due to a decline in male hormone (androgens) levels, primarily testosterone. From the age of 30 testosterone levels decrease about 1% per year. During this decline the body changes occur gradually and may be accompanied by symptoms similar to those of menopause.

ANDROPAUSE SYMPTOMS

- Weight gain
- Accelerated ageing of the heart
- Increased risk of cancer
- Increase in LDL cholesterol
- Osteoporosis
- Changes in attitudes and moods
- Irritability
- Depression
- Insomnia
- Lack of sex drive
- Erectile dysfunction or decreased strength of orgasm
- Increased fatigue
- Decreased energy and strength
- Loss of eagerness and enthusiasm
- Decreased mental acuity and loss of memory
- Increased body fat
- Rapidly falling level of fitness and decrease in muscle mass

- Decreased physical agility
- Stiffness and pain in the muscles and joints
- Some even experience sweating and hot flushes at night.

HOW DO YOU GET ANDROPAUSE?

- Excess alcohol intake
- Smoking
- Overweight and obesity
- Infections
- Stress
- Vasectomy
- Inactivity and lack of exercise

GET RID OF IT

Andropause is a true clinical entity that can be successfully and safely treated.

Too much estrogen and not enough testosterone, plummeting DHEA levels and reducing HGH levels are all correctable.

First, the hormone levels need to be established by blood or saliva tests. Often, increased estrogen levels accompany low testosterone levels. This information is important to ensure testosterone replacement is appropriate for him.

Men you need to:

- Lose weight – decrease body fat and increase muscle mass
- Exercise
- Avoid bread, sugar, alcohol
- Natural DHEA, natural testosterone and/or HGH.

MORE SEX, STAMINA AND SANITY

The most convenient form of administration of testosterone replacement for men is a troche or transdermal cream. Capsules and other oral preparations can be toxic to the liver.

Studies have shown increased libido, sexual enjoyment and function with testosterone replacement. Strength may improve without exercise, but there is a marked improvement with exercise.

Lean body mass increases and fat mass reduces. Bone density increases. Improving testosterone levels decreases heart attacks and strokes and improves blood flow, reducing angina. Diabetes can be improved with greater insulin resistance and decreased medication. There is a positive effect on brain function. Depression can improve with reduction of antidepressants and there may be a case for optimising testosterone levels before reaching for the antidepressants.

LOSE THE BEER GUT

Julian Whitaker MD, a nationally recognized pioneer in wellness and alternative medicine states, male testosterone levels start to slowly decrease beginning around age 30, then more rapidly around age 60. Testosterone is responsible for the development of bone and lean muscle mass in men. When this hormone's level declines, there is a loss of muscle strength and endurance during physical activities, a lowered metabolic rate and an accompanying accumulation of body fat. Studies have shown a direct correlation between testosterone levels and abdominal fat.

Testosterone is also involved in blood sugar control. Decreased levels of the hormone are associated with increased insulin output, a risk factor for the development of diabetes and a contributing factor in obesity. Decreased testosterone levels can lead to an increase in blood levels of the hormones: adrenaline and cortisol. If this state occurs for an extended period of time, the thyroid can be affected, which may slow down metabolism and lead to an accumulation of body fat.

CANCER WHERE IT HURTS

Testosterone should not be replaced above the physiologic range i.e. the range that is considered normal for a man. Prostate cancer is always of concern in men with who take testosterone supplemention as is of similar concern as breast cancer in women who take estrogen supplementation. However, there is no evidence to date that there is an increased incidence of prostate cancer with testosterone replacement. Actually, the reverse may be the case. It is important that a man starting testosterone replacement should routinely be monitored for prostate cancer by their doctor and early cancers may well be detected and effectively treated. Men with established prostate cancer are often advised not to undergo testosterone supplements.

A loss of testosterone in men may lead to osteoporosis. This may be prevented or treated with testosterone or even natural progesterone. Progesterone does not have feminising effects and will accomplish similar bone-building benefits as testosterone.

For more information visit: www.redwoodnhrt.com.au
or call 1300 304 638

PROSTATE CANCER

1 in 11 Australian men have a chance of developing prostate cancer 1 in 78 men have a chance of dying from it. It is the most common cancer in men, making up 23% of all cancers in Australia. One in four American men now has prostate cancer by age 50. 38,000 men have their prostates removed by surgery or radiation 40,000 men die from prostate cancer each year.

A belief, now outdated, was that testosterone was the culprit causing prostate cancer. Testosterone does NOT cause prostate cancer. If this were true 19 and 20-year old males would be developing prostate cancer as these are the individuals with the highest levels. This is obviously not the case. There is no firm evidence that testosterone causes prostate cancer, in fact, it appears the same hormone that causes breast cancer is the actual culprit. The most aggressive prostate cancers are correlated with levels of testosterone that are too low and estrogen levels that are too high. Sound familiar?

Estrogen is the main contributor to prostate cancer. It is actually the incomplete breakdown of estrogen in the liver. This produces 16-hydroxyestrone that is proven to cause prostate cancer.

Obesity, high alcohol consumption, xeno-estrogens and stress all increase estrogen in men.

A CANCEROUS PROSTATE

An enlarged prostate and hence prostate cancer can be easily screened for by a blood test, urine test and the old fashion manual test with a rubber glove.

The blood test is known as a PSA (prostate-specific antigen) test. A score greater than 2 mg/ml, could indicate a prostate problem or the early stages of prostate cancer.

A urine test can determine the ratio of 2- and 16- hydroxyestrones in men and also women. Too much 16- metabolite means that your liver is not effectively eliminating estrogen and you are at an increased risk for prostate and breast cancer.

KEEPING THE PROSTATE HEALTHY

DIET – Eat cruciferous vegetables (broccoli, cabbage). The phyto-chemicals in these cruciferous vegetables have been shown to beneficially affect the body's hormonal and detoxification systems. Epidemiological studies have supported the health benefits of consuming these vegetables. Eat tomatoes as they contain lycopene that assists in reducing the risk of prostate cancer.

INDOLE 3 CARBINOL – which prevents the conversion of testosterone to estrogen, therefore, inhibiting the formation of 16-hydroxyestrone.

DIM (diindolylmethane) has been shown to help regulate and promote a more efficient metabolism of estrogen an optimal ratio of estrogen metabolites important for male as well as female health.

VITAMIN D – Vitamin D deficiency has been strongly linked with prostate and breast cancer. Supplements are available if necessary or good old sun exposure without sunscreen will help.

NATURAL PROGESTERONE – Progesterone may also be helpful for men. Read on.

PROGESTERONE AND PROSTATE

The most exciting information available to date has to do with progesterone's ability to PREVENT and REVERSE many cancers. The newer studies as we have discussed show that estrogen, specifically estradiol, does not increase the risk for breast cancer but it actually CAUSES breast cancer AND prostate cancer.

Males also produce progesterone, although about half as much as females do. Progesterone prevents the body from converting testosterone to di-hydro testosterone. It does this by inhibiting the enzyme 5-alpha reductase. Progesterone inhibits 5-alpha-reductase far more effectively than any of the other herbal treatments.

For more information visit: www.redwoodnhrt.com.au
or call 1300 304 638

Part 4

HORMONE SELF EVALUATION TEST

The way you feel is the most important indicator that your hormones are not balanced and that they need to be addressed. You will spend an hour at most with your physician. That is not a lot of time to explain what is going on with your health on a daily basis. It is up to you to make a note of how you feel, when you feel different things and the severity of symptoms in relation to daily life. This will help you and your physician to work out exactly what is going on and how to address the problems. You should keep a simple journal of your periods and any other symptoms that are plaguing you. Here is a quick test that you can take to your physician to help identify what is happening with your hormones.

ARE YOU HORMONE DEFICIENT?

The following evaluation is personal and confidential. The purpose of this evaluation is for you to identify signs of a decline in hormones. You are encouraged to make your health care decisions in partnership with a qualified health care professional.

If you would like some assistance in understanding your evaluation and finding a qualified physician to help you with balancing your hormones please simply photocopy this hormone self evaluation test and fax to: 02 9389 4500 or mail to: PO Box 475, Double Bay, NSW 1360. You can also print this evaluation online at: www.redwoodnhrt.com.au

Read carefully through the list of symtoms in each section put a check mark next to each symptom that you have. In any group where you have two or more symptoms checked off, there's a good chance that you have the hormone imbalance represented by that group. It is also possible that you have a hormone deficiency in more than one category.

FOR THE WOMEN

SECTION 1: ESTROGEN DEFICIENCY

Vaginal dryness	
Painful intercourse	
Bladder infections	
Hot flushes	
Night sweats	
Fatigue	
Depression	
Incontinence	
Insomnia	
Decreased sexual response	
Foggy thinking	
Low bone density	
Heart palpitations	

SECTION 2: EXCESS ESTROGEN/ESTROGEN DOMINANCE

Puffiness and bloating	
Weight gain in hips	
Mood swings	
Anxiety and irritability	
Depression	
Frequent thrush	
Weepiness	
Carbohydrate craving (Sugar/Bread)	
Diminishes sex drive	
Breast tenderness	
Foggy thinking	
Fibroids	
Fibrocystic breasts	
Premenstrual headaches and migraines	
Heavy bleeding	

SECTION 3: PROGESTERONE DEFICIENCY

PMS	
Irregular periods	
Night sweats	
Low bone density	
Early miscarriage	
Weepiness	
Insomnia	
Sore or swollen breasts	
Headaches associated with your period	
Infertility	
Anxiety	

SECTION 4: EXCESS ANDROGENS (MALE HORMONES)

Acne	
Excessive hair on face and arms	
Thinning hair on head	
Ovarian cysts	
Infertility	
Pain when ovulating	
Unstable blood sugar	
Polycystic ovary syndrome (PCOS)	
Irritability	
Deepened voice	
Elevated cholesterol	
High blood pressure	

SECTION 5: THYROID DEFICIENCY

Fatigue, lack of energy	
Weight gain or difficulty losing weight	
Low body temperature	
Fluid retention	
Constipation	
Pale, dry skin	
Puffiness in face, hands and feet	
Depression, anxiety	
Irritabilty	
Intolerance to cold or heat	
Stiffness of the joints	

SECTION 6: MELATONIN DEFICIENCY

Insomnia	
Suffer from jet lag when travelling	
Feel un-rested upon waking in the morning	
Tendency to be over-heated	
Shift work	

FOR THE MEN

SECTION 1: TESTOSTERONE DEFICIENCY

Weight loss	
Loss of muscle	
Diminished sex drive	
Enlarged breasts	
Lower stamina	
Weaker erections	
Fatigue	
Depression	
Gallbladder problems	

SECTION 2: EXCESS ESTROGEN

Hair loss	
Headaches	
Breast enlargement	
Weight gain	
Irritability	
Bloating and/or puffiness	

SECTION 3: THYROID DEFICIENCY

Fatigue, lack of energy	
Weight gain or difficulty losing weight	
Low body temperature	
Fluid retention	
Constipation	
Pale, dry skin	
Puffiness in face, hands and feet	
Depression, anxiety	
Irritability	
Intolerance to cold or heat	
Stiffness of the joints	

SECTION 4: MELATONIN DEFICIENCY

Insomnia	
Suffer from jet lag when travelling	
Feel un-rested upon waking in the morning	
Tendency to be easily over-heated	
Shift work	

WHAT DOES THIS MEAN?

FOR THE WOMEN

SECTION 1: ESTROGEN DEFICIENCY

Estrogen deficiency is the most common hormone imbalance in menopausal women. Helpful changes for an estrogen deficiency include: diet, exercise some women may even need a little bit of natural estrogen.

SECTION 2: EXCESS ESTROGEN/ESTROGEN DOMINANCE

Too much estrogen can often be the cause of your current supplementation. Helpful changes to correct excess estrogen include: Stop conventional synthetic hormone replacement and investigate the ratio of progesterone to estrogen in your body. An estrogen "blocker" supplementation such as Indole 3 Carbinol may also be useful.

SECTION 3: PROGESTERONE DEFICIENCY

This hormone imbalance is the most common deficiency in women of all ages. Helpful changes for a progesterone deficiency include: diet, avoiding synthetic HRT or "the pill" and natural progesterone cream perhaps.

SECTION 4: EXCESS ANDROGENS (DHEA & TESTOSTERONE)

Excess androgens in woman can be quite easily rebalanced. Too much sugar and simple carbohydrates in the diet most often cause of this hormone imbalance. Helpful changes for correcting excess androgens include: reducing sugar and carbohydrate intake and a full hormone assessment to determine other sex hormones.

SECTION 5: THYROID DEFICIENCY

A thyroid imbalance is very common in women and men of all ages. Helpful changes to correct a thyroid deficiency include: diet, T3, T4 or a combination of both or natural thyroid extract.

SECTION 6: MELATONIN DEFICIENCY

A melatonin deficiency can be easily corrected with melatonin capsules or cream.

FOR THE MEN

SECTION 1: TESTOSTERONE DEFICIENCY

This deficiency is the most common in men over the age of 40. Helpful changes for a testosterone deficiency include: diet, muscle-building exercise, such as weights natural hormone supplementation with DHEA and/or testosterone.

SECTION 2: EXCESS ESTROGEN

Excess estrogen in men can be corrected and rebalanced. Helpful changes for men with excess estrogen include: diet, exercise and natural hormone supplementation such as DHEA and/or testosterone or estrogen "blocker" such as Indole 3 Carbinol or DIM.

SECTION 3: THYROID DEFICIENCY

A thyroid imbalance is very common in women and men of all ages. Helpful changes to correct a thyroid deficiency include: diet, T3, T4 or a combination of both or natural thyroid extract.

SECTION 4 = MELATONIN DEFICIENCY

A melatonin deficiency can be easily corrected with melatonin capsules or cream.

If you would like some assistance in understanding your evaluation and finding a qualified physician to help you with balancing your hormones please simply photocopy this hormone self evaluation test and fax to: 02 9389 4500 or mail to: PO Box 475, Double Bay, NSW 1360. You can also print this evaluation online at: www.redwoodnhrt.com.au

GET YOURSELF TESTED

There are many options for testing that can help determine your hormone levels. There are tests for just about every function of your body and they can act as useful instruments for you and your physician to determine your starting point and your progress. Some tests are rebatable from Medicare or private health insurance and some need to be self-funded.

Saliva Tests – ordered by you or your physician

Blood Tests – ordered by your physician

Urine Tests – ordered by you or your physician

Blood Spot Tests – ordered by you or your physician

Bone Density Tests – ordered by you or your physician

SALIVA HORMONE TEST

This measurement technique does not have the same standards as blood testing, but it is convenient and some argue that it is more accurate than blood testing.

Your saliva contains free hormones that can be easily measured to give an accurate picture of those hormones available to your tissues. Saliva tests measure the amount of hormone that your body is actually experiencing.

It is highly recommended to get a saliva test for a base line level to start with; repeating the test in 2 to 3 months. This way you will be able to evaluate if your natural hormone replacement therapy has affected your levels. It is then recommended to repeat the test once a year thereafter.

Comparing your hormone levels to the normal range for your age will help you and your doctor in evaluating how your natural hormone replacement therapy will or has influenced your hormone levels.

Saliva tests can measure estriol, estradiol, estrone, progesterone, testosterone, cortisol, DHEA and melatonin.

BLOOD TEST

This measurement technique has the advantage of widespread established technology and standards. Most published studies that document the safety and efficacy of proper hormone replacement therapy rely on blood tests rather than saliva testing.

There is a difference of opinion among experts regarding whether blood levels provide an accurate reflection of the amount of hormone in the tissues in comparison to saliva and urine. While some physicians advocate blood testing as the most accurate, another equally knowledgeable group of physicians argues that saliva or urine testing is much more accurate.

It is important to remember that different laboratories have different standards. For example, the "normal range" advised by Pathology Lab A may be very different to Pathology Lab B. Standards from one laboratory should not be used to evaluate testing by another source. In addition, it is impossible to give a representative sample of all the possible optimal or even average scores because these figures change based on age, pregnancy status, menopausal status, the particular day within each woman's menstrual cycle and time of day.

BONE DENSITY TEST

The best test to determine whether you have bone loss is the bone mineral density test (BMD).

Currently the most reliable and accurate test for measuring bone density is the DEXA (dual energy x-ray absorptiometry). This test helps detect early bone loss and is widely available worldwide.

The DEXA test will give you results as 2 scores -
T score: This compares your bone density with that of an average young adult of the same sex
T score = 0: means your bones are the same density as the average younger population
T score = above 1: means your bones are denser than the average younger population

T score = below 0: means your bones are less dense than the average younger population

You will also receive a Z score. The Z score compares your bone density with the average of people in your age group and gender.

Z score = 0 means your bones are average for your age.

Z score = below 0: means your bones are below average density

Z score = above 0: means your bones are above average density for your age

Z score = below –2: means you are losing bone more rapidly than your peers, so you need to monitor treatment carefully.

Results below 0 are indicative that you require treatment and your options need to be discussed with your doctor.

Part 5

THE RIGHT CHOICE FOR YOU

The decision for you to take control of your life and take natural hormones is a personal one.

The correct combination of hormones needed for your natural hormone treatment will be determined by taking into account the following;

- Your age
- Your body weight, size and shape
- Your medical history of your health problems and concerns
- Your bone density level
- Your symptoms and expectations
- Your results of hormone levels in blood and salivary tests

I encourage you to evaluate your individual needs, quality of life and your risk factors before you make an informed decision.

WHERE DO I GET THE REAL NATURAL HORMONES?

A compounding pharmacy acquires the pure pharmaceutical grade hormones and compounds them into the form ordered by your doctor. An experienced compounding pharmacy can make your natural hormone program very customized and personalised.

Products offered by health food stores and alternative practitioners provide people with a variety of natural options usually from herb or plant source but they CANNOT provide natural hormones. Naturopaths, Homeopaths and Herbalists have evolved and their remedies are more substantiated and better accepted but can provide only alternative, herbal products. However, the products from a compounding pharmacy, by a prescription of a medical physician are different in several ways.

First, the dose provided by a pharmacy requires a prescription by law. Health food store products do not. They have a "one size fits all" approach and most often the dose is insufficient in producing a measurable difference in the body. Think about it – if it requires a prescription you can't buy it off the shelf.

Second, the products from a compounding pharmacy use ingredients of a pure pharmaceutical grade that are regulated heavily and "micronised". Micronised indicates that the product is a fine grain that will be well absorbed. This ensures you are getting the maximum benefits and also reducing the waste as it progresses through your digestive system in the case of oral preparations.

Third, the natural hormones offered by a compounding pharmacy can be prescribed as long-acting or sustained release. This helps the body have a more balanced hormone level instead of the highs and lows that came with quick acting, quickly absorbed or poorly absorbed products. This is very important for thyroid medications in particular.

Last, but not least, a compounding pharmacy can work with your physician to customise an individual prescription for you. This alone provides lots of options for a personal natural hormone program. The compounding pharmacy can combine multiple hormones if you require them to. This will help to reduce the cost, the time and the fuss.

Ask your physician about natural hormones and then get in touch with a compounding pharmacy - one that is committed to providing high quality compounded medications in the dosage form and strength prescribed by the physician. Through the triad relationship of patient, physician and pharmacist, all three can work together to solve unique medical problems. If your doctor would like to find out any information regarding Redwood or Natural Hormone Replacement please ask them to call Redwood on 1300 304 638

WHEN DO I TAKE NATURAL HRT?

As you have learned there are many hormones that can help you. Discuss your best options with your physician. Here are a few guidelines that may help you.

Ideally, the best way to take natural hormones is to take one half of the daily dose every 12 hours for oral, sublingual and topical doses.

However, this is not always the case.

- Estrogen for night sweats is best to take with your evening meal.
- Testosterone sublingual for libido is best to take 2 hours before bedtime.
- DHEA is best taken after breakfast.
- Progesterone is best to take at bedtime.
- Melatonin is best taken on an empty stomach 30 minutes to 2 hours before going to bed.

EASY DOES IT

The key to hormonal health is balance. Natural hormone treatment should be prescribed in the smallest effective doses in an individual plan and supervised by a qualified physician.

With the proper physiological doses of natural hormones you can regain your youthful zeal and energy and get rid of your health problems but too much or too little will be to the detriment of your health and your wallet.

Dosing hormones should be an individual decision. The response to natural hormone therapy can be varied. It can be due to differences in the absorption of the hormone. Each patient can respond uniquely to a given dose.

The prescribed dosage should be based on each patient's medical and family history, current health status, personal habits, symptoms and priorities. The best plan of attack is to start conservatively and monitor changes and progress to achieve the right dose for you.

GIVE ME THE BEST CHOICE

The best choice is the one that works for you. Natural hormone compounds give you that choice. Whether you need natural progesterone, estrone, estriol, estradiol, DHEA, testosterone, pregnenolone, indole 3 carbinol, DIM, human growth hormone, melatonin or a combination of the above, compounded natural hormone formulation can help you.

Just about anything can be made just to suit you! Everyone is different. So what is best for one, may not be best for another. Sometimes you need to try 2 or 3 different delivery systems until you find what works best for you.

Have your medications the way you like them:

- Capsules – oral
- Troches – sublingual
- Creams – transdermal
- Gels and Oils – transdermal
- Suppositories – rectal
- Pessaries – vaginal

If you can't swallow medications you can use a troche or cream. If you're allergic to dyes have your medication without! If you want it sweet, just add flavour! Sounds more like a restaurant! If you would like more information visit www.redwoodnhrt.com.au or call 1300 304 638.

NOT TOO PRICEY

Compounding may not cost more than a conventional or synthetic medication. The cost depends on the type of delivery method, individual amounts of ingredients required and the complexity of preparing the medication.

A specialised compounding pharmacy has access to pure grade quality ingredients, which dramatically lowers overall costs and allows them to be very competitive with commercially manufactured products. This also ensures you are "getting what you paid for".

You can get a rebate from private health insurers for natural hormone replacement therapy. You will need to check with your private health insurance provider for the rebate available to you.

I DON'T HAVE A DOCTOR WHO WILL LISTEN!

Natural Hormone prescription compounding is a rapidly growing component of many doctor's practices, but in today's world of aggressive marketing by big drug manufacturers, some may not realise all of the natural hormone options that are available. In many cases you will know more than your doctor.

If your doctor will not listen and you need to find a doctor in your area that will prescribe the kind of natural hormones you want and need, Redwood can help you. Redwood has a comprehensive list of doctors worldwide who are familiar with natural hormone replacement. To find a doctor who will listen and regain your sanity call 1300 304 638.

WHAT OTHERS ARE SAYING ABOUT BIO-IDENTICAL HORMONES?

"For me, natural hormone replacement is a safer choice than synthetic hormones. For years on the synthetic hormones, I suffered from low energy and severe night sweats. The natural hormones are natural to my body and have help relieve those symptoms and more! I feel great!"
Mrs. K Brown, NSW

"I was starting to wonder what was wrong with me. I was so irritable and impatient. I couldn't understand how my family could live with me. But now I feel great...like my normal self. My husband is happy again and doesn't threaten to move out of the house once a month!"
Mrs. S Tester, NSW

"I didn't have any menopausal symptoms, I felt truly blessed but cardiovascular disease and breast cancer run in my family. I wanted to protect myself from these diseases and refuse to take pregnant horses urine. I couldn't believe my luck when a friend told me about the natural hormones. Thanks to a doctor who finally listened, natural hormones, exercise and my trusty vitamins I feel even more fantastic and I rest easy knowing I am doing everything I can to protect myself."
Ms. D McClelland, QLD

"Since the menopause I have had fluid retention, bloating and insomnia. But since my doctor prescribed me natural estrogen and progesterone combined this has all gone away. After some months on the treatment my libido and sexual enjoyment is improving."
Mrs. C Whalley, NSW

"Thank you so much, the cream has made such a wonderful difference."
Mrs. C Ward, SA

"Since starting on the Pill in my early 20's I have found myself on the synthetic hormone merry-go-round. For years my regular GP's and even

my gynecologist could never explain why I felt so horrible or offer me a solution to the effects of those synthetic drugs. At last a doctor introduced me to the natural hormone sand for the first time in a long time I feel in control and I feel I'm giving my body what it really needs".
Mrs. J Roberts, NSW

"The natural hormones have benefited me by making me feel as I did before menopause began. I feel confident and more energetic... I do not have hot flushes anymore and my night sweats have gone completely. I want sex more often and my husband is happy with me again!"
Mrs. L Trojanowski, NSW

"Since... taking the natural progesterone for my monthly hormone hell I have felt more energetic. I am less 'PMSy'. ... my carbohydrate craving has decreased and I have managed to lose weight too!."
Ms. K Hill, New Zealand

"As a compounding pharmacist, I hope all women will read this book and more doctors can gain understanding of the information presented in it. As for the thousands of women I know to be using natural hormone replacement therapy, I have never before in over 20 years of practice received so much appreciative mail and letters of thanks from patients whose lives have been turned around by this therapy."
Mr. D Knowles, NSW

"HOW DHEA REPLACEMENT THERAPY HAS CHANGED MY LIFE"

Daniel, a 28-year-old from South Australia suffered from chronic fatigue syndrome (CFS) for over two years. The illness brought along many unpleasant side effects Daniel could not live his active and enthusiastic lifestyle anymore. He felt he was deteriorating quickly as the illness progressed. Then he discovered the cause and also the cure for this sickness...

"Up until about two years ago, I was a normal, happy and active person. I have always loved the outdoors. Then I developed

Chronic Fatigue Syndrome and everything went downhill from there..."

How did the illness affect Daniel's life?

"CFS damaged me, it virtually knocked me out and life was not normal anymore. I was lethargic and got puffed out after just 300 yards of walking. Everything was very exhausting.

Every morning I would be sick. I didn't know why this was happening to me. I just got used to it. Throughout the day I did not have the energy to do the things I used to do, I was too exhausted to perform in any type of activity, even taking my girlfriend shopping was not possible anymore.

I began talking like an old man – well that was exactly how I felt. I couldn't even do work for prolonged periods of time as that was even exhausting..."

Clearly life could not continue like this, Daniel had tried many types of medication – all without any sign of improvement.

"I undertook many tests; however, everything appeared to be fine. Then, about 1 year ago, I learned about Hormone Replacement Therapies. Although one assumes this is usually for older people, I decided to have my hormone levels checked out, after all, I did feel like I was 70 or 80 years of age! When my doctor, Dr Baran, checked my DHEA levels we found out that they were incredibly low. Dr Baran explained that low levels of DHEA could be the cause of my health problems."

"First I thought it was a lot of garbage, I had tried so many things along the way, including synthetic hormone replacement products and homeopathic remedies such as a DHEA mouth spray and pharmaceutical products. None of these did anything for me. But I had come to a point where I was prepared to try anything, if only it would make the slightest difference.

Daniel started applying DHEA cream daily. "It was amazing stuff. How I lived with it (CFS) for two years is beyond me. I have never felt better than I do now!"

Once Daniel started to use the DHEA, he began to feel normal again, for the first time in the last couple of years.

"I felt still do feel, so energetic. The amazing thing is that it only took two days for the DHEA treatment to take effect. I get out of bed in the morning and feel fine. I can begin my day without hours of sickness, nausea and struggling. I am fully awake all the time and not lethargic like before."

Apart from restoring his energy, the DHEA treatment has improved other areas of Daniel's health.

"I sometimes used to get grumpy. Like a woman with PMS, I'd feel really moody. It was then that I knew that the problem had to be hormonal. Since applying the cream, my mood swings have disappeared."

"I never used to be able to sleep; I was tossing and turning all night, Low DHEA levels must have contributed to this, too. Depression and back pain, which I used to suffer from regularly in the past, have gone. It seems as if restoring my hormone levels has rebalanced my whole life."

Mr. Daniel Sarantidis, SA

DON'T JUST TAKE OUR WORD FOR IT

You have so many valuable resources available to you. Books, Internet, seminars, courses and talking to others are all available to you. We implore you to find out everything you need to know to feel comfortable that natural hormones are for you.

READ AND LEARN

A Woman's Guide to Natural Hormones by Christine Conrad,

Hormone Replacement Therapy, Yes or No by Betty Kamen M.D

Maximize Your Vitality & Potency: For Men Over 40 by Jonathan V. Wright. M.D. & Lane Lenard,

Natural Hormone Replacement Therapy; by Jonathan V. Wright, M.D. & John Morgenthaler

PMS: The Essential Guide to Treatment Options by Dr. Katharina Dalton

Stopping the Clock by Dr Robert Goldman

The Anti-Ageing Diet by Brian Sher

The Hormone Solution by Thierry Hertoghe, M.D

The Testosterone Syndrome: Reversing the Male Menopause by Eugene Shippen, M.D. & William Fryer

The HRT Solution: Optimizing Your Hormone Potential, by Marla Ahlgrimm, RPh & John M. Kells

What Your Doctor May Not Tell You About PreMenopause by Dr. John Lee

Women's Bodies, Women's Wisdom by Christiane Northrup, M.D.

SURF AND LEARN

Dr John Lee – Natural Progesterone – www.johnleemd.com

Redwood – www.redwoodnhrt.com.au

Redwood Anti-Ageing – www.redwoodantiageing.com

American Academy of Anti-Ageing Medicine – www.worldhealth.net

ADVANCED SURFING

www.medline.com – Free online database of the National Library of Medicine. PubMed, by the NLM, is completely free extremely easy to search. See also the National Library of Medicine's extensive links to journals that offer online full-text articles

www.whi.org – The latest findings and information regarding the Women's Health Initiative Study.

www.thelancet.com – Lancet Journal Website. The world's most prestigious independent journal of general medicine. The Lancet does not have the bias against publishing well-designed trials of natural HRT, clinical nutrition, herbal medicine, or alternative therapies unlike other journals. There are many free educational articles on this site.

www.nature.com/medicalresearch – Register online to receive medical updates on topics of interest. This site has many medical articles and links to medical journals.

REFERENCES

"AACE Medical Guidelines for Clinical Practice for the Evaluation and Treatment of Hyperthyroidism and Hypothyroidism" *Endocrine Practice*, Vol. 8, No. 6, Nov/Dec 2002.

"Effects of Conjugated Equine Estrogen in Postmenopausal Women with Hysterectomy" *American Medical Association*, 2004. Reprinted with permission *JAMA* , Vol 291. No14, 2004; 1701.

"Hormonal regulation of the differentiation of rat preadipocytes." *Nutr Rev.* 1988; 46: 235-36.

"Osteoporosis contribution to modern management." The proceedings of a Symposium held at the XVIIth Congress of Rheumatology, Rio de Janeiro, September 1989. Ed. B.E.C. Nordin. Novartis, New Jersey: The Parthenon Publishing Group, 1990. "Report International Health Foundation": ref 10 A 32 b.

"Women seeking safe alternatives to synthetic HRT: Natural HRT alternatives based on science not guesswork" US Newswire August 5, 2002 p1008217n0665.

Abbasi, A., et al. "Association of dehydroepiandrosterone sulfate, body composition physical fitness in independent community-dwelling older men and women." *J Am Geriatr Soc.* 1998; 46 (3): 263-73.

Abdu, T. A., et al. "Coronary risk in growth hormone deficient hypopituitary adults: increased predicted risk is due largely to lipid profile abnormalities." *Clin Endocrinol (Oxf).* 2001; 55 (2): 209-16.

Abrahamssons, L., et al. "Catabolic effects and the influence on hormonal variables under treatment with gynodian-depot or DHEA oenanthate." *Maturitas.* 1981; 3: 225-34.

Adami, H. O., et al. "Survival and age at diagnosis in breast cancer." *N Engl J Med.* 1987; 316 752.

Adami, H. O., et al. "The effect of female sex hormones on cancer survival." *JAMA.* 1990; 263 (16): 2189-93.

Adlin, E. V., et al. "Bone mineral density in postmenopausal women treated with L-thyroxine." *Am J Med.* 1991; 90 (3): 360-66.

Aiman, J., Brenner, P.F., MacDonald, P.C. Androgen and estrogen production in elderly men with gynecomastia and testicular atrophy after mumps orchitis. *J. Clin. Endocrinol. Metab.* 1980 Feb; 50(2): 380-6.

Akbulut, K. G., et al. "The effects of melatonin on humoral immune responses of young and aged rats." *Immunol Invest.* 2001; 30 (1): 17-20.

Akumabor, P. N., "Is pre-treatment testosterone a prognostic factor in prostate cancer?" *Cent Afr J Med.* 1993; 39 (8): 170-72.

Alba-Roth, J., et al. "Arginine stimulates growth hormone secretion by suppressing endogenous somatostatin secretion." *J Clin Endocrinol Metab.* 1988; 57:1186-88.

Alberg, A. J., et al. "Serum dehydroepiandrosterone and dehydroepiandrosterone sulfate and the subsequent risk of developing colon cancer." *Cancer Epidemiol Biomarkers Prev.* 2000; 9 (5): 517-21.

Alexander, G. M., et al. "Androgen-behavior correlations in hypogonadal men and eugonadal men. I. Mood and response to auditory sexual stimuli." *Horm Behav.* 1997; 31 (2): 110-19.

Alexandersen, P., et al. "The relationship of natural androgens to coronary heart disease in males: a review." *Atherosclerosis.* 1996; 125 (1): 1-13.

Allen, R. C., et al. "Insulin-like growth factor and growth hormone secretion in juvenile chronic arthritis." *Ann Rheum Dis.* 1991; 50 (9): 602-6.

Angeli, A., "Effects of long-term; low-dose; time-specified melatonin administration on endocrine and cardiovascular variables in adult men." *J Pineal Res.* 1990; 9 (2): 113-24.

Antonijevic, I. A., et al. "Modulation of the sleep electroencephalogram by estrogen replacement in postmenopausal women." *Am J Obstet Gynecol.* 2000; 182 (2): 277-82.

Aoyama, H., et al. "Effects of melatonin on genetic hypercholesterolemia in rats." *Atherosclerosis.* 1988; 69: 269-72.

Applezwig, M. H., et al. "The pituitary-adrenocortical system in avoidance learning." *Psychol Rep.* 1955; 1: 417-20.

Arendt J, Aldhous M and Marks V. Alleviation of jet-lag by melatonin: Preliminary results of controlled double-blind trial. *Brit Med J.* 292:1170, 1986. Arem, Ridha MD. The Thyroid Solution, Ballantine Books, 1999

Argente, J., et al. "Multiple endocrine abnormalities of the growth hormone and insulin-like growth factor axis in patients with anorexia nervosa: effect of short long-term weight recuperation." *J Clin Endocrinol Metab.* 1997; 82 (7): 2084-92.

Arlt, W, et al. "DHEA replacement in women with adrenal insufficiencypharmacokinetics, bioconversion and clinical effects on well-being, sexuality and cognition." *Endocr Res.* 2000; 26 (4): 505-11.

Arlt, W., et al. "DHEA replacement in women with adrenal insufficiencypharmacokinetics, bioconversion and clinical effects on well-being, sexuality and cognition." *Endocr Res.* 2000; 26 (4): 505-11.

Arlt, W., et al. "Dehydroepiandrosterone replacement in women with adrenal insufficiency." *N Engl J Med.* 1999; 341 (14): 1013-20.

Armario, A., et al. "Influence of intensity and duration of exposure to various stressors on serum TSH and GH levels in adult male rats." *Life Sciences.* 1989; 44 (3): 215-27.

Arthur, J. R., et al. "Selenium deficiency thyroid hormone metabolism and thyroid hormone deiodinases." *Am J Clin Nutr Suppl.* 1993; 57: 236S-99.

Arver, S., et al. "Long-term efficacy and safety of a permeation-enhanced testosterone transdermal system in hypogonadal men." *Clin Endocrinol (Oxf).* 1997; 47 (6): 727-37.

Arvers, S., et al. "Improvement of sexual function in testosterone deficient men treated for 1 year with a permeation enhanced testosterone transdermal system.") *Urol.* 1996; 155 (5): 1604-8.

Aschoff, L. *Lectures on Pathology.* New York: Ed Hoeber, 1924; 5: 101.

Asthana, S., et al. "High-dose estradiol improves cognition for women with AD: results of a randomized study." *Neurology.* 2001; 57 (4): 605-12.

Astrom, C., et al. "Growth hormone-deficient young adults have decreased deep sleep." *Neuroendocrinology.* 1990; 51 (1): 82-84.

Astrom, C., et al. "The influence of growth hormone on sleep in adults with growth hormone deficiency." *Clin Endocrinol (Oxf).* 1990; 33 (4): 495-500.

Astrup A, Buemann B, Toubro S, Ranneries C, Raben A. Low resting metabolic rate in subjects predisposed to obesity: a role for thyroid status. Am J Clin Nutr 1996;63(6):879-873.

Backstrom. T., et al. "Ovarian steroid hormones." *Acta Obstet Gynecol Scand Suppl.* 1985; 130: 19.

Badwe, R. A., et al. "Serum progesterone at the time of surgery and survival in women with premenopausal operable breast cancer." *Eur J Cancer.* 1994; 30A (4): 445-48.

Barnes, B. O. "Etiology and treatment of lowered resistance to upper respiratory infections." *Fed Proc.* 1953; 12 (1): 24.

Barnes, B. O. "Role of the thyroid in infectious diseases." *Am Med Ass An Meeting.* 1965 June 24; New York.

Barnes, B. O., et al. *Hypothyroidism: The unsuspected Illness.* New York: Harper & Row Publishers, 1976;155-96.

Barrett-Connor, E. "A prospective study of DHEAs, mortality and cardiovascular disease." *N Engl J Med.* 1986; 315 (24): 1519-24.

Barrett-Connor, E., "A prospective study of DHEAs, mortality and cardiovascular disease." *N Engl J Med.* 1986; 315 (24): 1519-24.

Barrett-Connor, E., et al. "DHEA, DHEAs, obesity, waist-hip ratio non-insulin-dependent diabetes in postmenopausal women: the Rancho Bernardo Study." *J Clin Endocrinol Metab.* 1996; 81 (1): 59-64.

Barrett-Connor, E., et al. "Endogenous levels of dehydroepiandrosterone sulfate, but not other sex hormones, are associated with depressed mood in older women: the Rancho Bernardo Study." *J Am Geriatr Soc.* 1999; 47 (6): 685-91.

Barrett-Connor, E., et al. "Endogenous sex hormones and cardiovascular disease in men- A prospective population-based study." *Circulation.* 1988; 78: 539-45.

Barrett-Connor, E., et al. "The epidemiology of DHEAs and cardiovascular disease." *Ann NY Acad Sci.* 1995; 774: 259-70.

Barry, S., et al. "Neuroendocrine challenge tests in depression: a study of growth hormone, TRH and cortisol release. " *J Affect Disord.* 1990; 18 (4): 229-34.

Bartsch, C., et al. "Melatonin in cancer patients and in tumor-bearing animals." *Adv Exp Med Biol.* 1999; 467: 247-64.

Bastianetto, S., et al. "Dehydroepiandrosterone (DHEA) protects hippocampal cells from oxidative stress-induced damage." *Brain Res Mol Brain Res.* 1999; 66 (1-2): 35-41.

Bauer, M., et al. "Psychological and endocrine abnormalities in refugees from East Germany: Part I. Prolonged stress, psychopathology hypothalamic-pituitary-thyroid axis activity." *Psychiatry Res.* 1994; 51 (1): 61-73.

Baulieu, E. E., et al. "Dehydroepiandrosterone (DHEA), DHEA sulfate aging: contribution of the DHEAge Study to a sociobiomedical issue." *Proc Natl Acad Sci USA.* 2000; 97 (8): 4279-84.

Beer, N. A., et al. "Dehydroepiandrosterone reduces plasma plasminogen activator inhibitor type 1 and tissue plasminogen activator antigen in men." *Am J Med Sci.* 1996; 311 (5): 205-10.

Beisel, W. R., et al. "Interrelations between adrenocortical functions and infectious illness." *N Engl Med.* 1969; 280: 541-46.

Bender, C. E. "The value of corticosteroids in the treatment of infectious mononucleosis." *J AMA.* 1967; 199:539-31.

Bengtsson, B. A., et al. "Treatment of adults with growth hormone deficiency with recombinant human GH." *J Clin Endocrinol Metab.* 1993;76:309-17.

Bennett, R. M., et al. "Low levels of somatomedin C in patients with the fibromyalgia syndrome. A possible link between sleep and muscle pain." *Arthritis Rheum.* 1992; 35 (10): 1113-16.

Bernini, G. P., et al. "Influence of endogenous androgens on carotid wall in postmenopausal women." *Menopause.* 2001; 8 (1): 43-50.

Berrino, F., et al. "Reducing bioavailable sex hormones through a comprehensive change in diet: the diet and androgens (DIANA) randomized trial." *Cancer Epidemiol Biomarkers Prev.* 2001; 10 (1): 25-33.

Bhasin, S., et al. "Testosterone dose-response relationships in healthy young men." *Am J Physiol Endocrinol Metab.* 2001; 281 (6): E1172-81.

Bitran, D., et al. "Anxiolytic effect of progesterone is mediated by the neurosteroid allopregnenolone at brain GABA receptors." *J Neuroendocrinol.* 1995; 7 (3): 171-77.

Bixo, M., et al. "Progesterone distribution in the brain of the PMSG treated female rat." *Acta Physiol Scand.* 1984; 122: 355.

Blache, D., et al. "Inhibition of sexual behaviour and the luteinizing hormone surge by intracerebral progesterone implants in the female sheep." *Brain Res.* 1996; 741 (1-2): 117-22.

Blaicher, W., et al. "Melatonin in postmenopausal females." *Arch Gynecol Obstet.* 2000; 263 (3): 116-18.

Bloch, M., et al. "Dehydroepiandrosterone treatment of midlife dysthymia." *Biol Psychiatry.* 1999; 45 (12): 1533-41.

Block, G., "Epidemiologic evidence regarding vitamin C and cancer." *Am J Clin Nutr.* 1991; 54: 13105-45.

Bogardus, G. M., et al. "Breast cancer and thyroid disease." *Surgery.* 1961; 49 (4): 461-68.

Boing, H., et al. "Regional nutritional pattern and cancer mortality in the Federal Republic of Germany." *Nutr Cancer.* 1985; 7 (3): 121-36.

Bolognia, J. L. "Aging skin." *Am J Med.* 1995; 98 (1A): 995-1035.

Boman, K., et al. "The influence of progesterone and androgens on the growth of endometrial carcinoma." *Cancer.* 1993; 71 (11): 3565-69.

Bonnet, K. A., et al. "Cognitive effects of DHEA replacement therapy." In *The Biological Role of DHEA*, eds. W. Regelson and M. Kalimi. Berlin: Walter de Gruyter & Co., 1990; 65-79.

Boone, J. B., Jr., et al. "Resistance exercise effects on plasma cortisol, testosterone and creatine kinase activity in anabolic-androgenic steroid users." *Int J Sports Med.* 1990; 11 (4): 293-97.

Bou-Holaigah, I., et al. "The relationship between neurally mediated hypotension and the chronic fatigue syndrome." *JAMA.* 1995; 274 (12): 961-67.

Boukhliq, R., et al. "Role of glucose, fatty acids and protein in regulation of testicular growth and secretion of gonadotropin, prolactin, somatotropin and insulin in the mature ram." *Reprod Fertil Dev.* 1997; 9 (5): 515-24.

Bourinbaiar, A. S., et al. "Pregnancy hormones, estrogen and progesterone, prevent HIV-1 synthesis in monocytes but not in lymphocytes." *Febs Lett.* 1992; 302 (3): 206-8.

Bradlow HL, et al. 16 a hydroxylation of estradiol: A possible risk marker for breast cancer. *Biochem Biophys Res Commun* 1986; 237: 138-151.

Brincat, M., et al. "Long-term effects of the menopause and sex hormones on skin thickness." *Br J Obstet Gynaecol.* 1985; 92: 256-59.

Bringhurst, E R., et al "Hormones of the mineral metabolism. Calcitonin." In *Williams' Endocrinology.* 9th ed., vol 24. Philadelphia: W. B. Saunders Company, 1998; 1164-66.

Brixen, K., et al. "A short course of recombinant human growth hormone treatment stimulates osteoblasts and activates bone remodeling in normal human volunteers." *J Bone Miner Res.* 1990; 5 (6): 609-18.

Browstein, David MD - The Miracle of Natural Hormones 3rd Edition - 2003

Brugger, P., et al. "Impaired nocturnal secretion of melatonin in coronary heart disease." *Lancet.* 1995; 345 (8962): 1408.

Bruno, O. D., et al. "Thyroid gland function and autoimmunity in children with alopecia universalis." *Medicine B Aires.* 1985; 45 (1): 25-28.

Buchanan, J. R., et al. "Effect of excess endogenous androgens on bone density in young women." *J Clin Endocrinol Metab.* 1988; 67 (5): 937.

Buckley, L. M., et al. "Effects of low dose corticosteroids on the bone mineral density of patients with rheumatoid arthritis." *J Rheumatol.* 1995; 22 (6): 1055-59.

Buckman R. & Dear W. "What you really need to know about hormone replacement therapy" Macmillan Canada 1999

Buiatti, F., et al. "A case-control of gastric cancer and diet in Italy: association with nutrients." *Int J Cancer.* 1990; 45: 899-901.

Bulbrook, R. D., et al. "Abnormal excretion of urinary steroids by women with early breast cancer." *Lancet.* 1962; 1238-40.

Bush, T. L., et al. "Cardiovascular mortality and noncontraceptive use of estrogen in women: Results from the lipid Research Clinics Program Follow-up Study." *Circulation.* 1987; 75: 1102-9.

Cagnacci, A., et al. "Different circulatory response to melatonin in postmenopausal women without and with hormone replacement therapy." *J Pineal Res.* 2000; 29 (3): 152-58.

Cagnaccid, A., et al. "Hypothermic effect of melatonin and nocturnal core body temperature decline are reduced in aged women." *J Appl Physiol.* 1995; 78 (1): 314-17.

Cai, X., et al. "High-fat diet increases the weight of rat ventral prostate." *Prostate.* 2001; 49 (1): 1-8.

Cai, X., et al. "Pilot study of dietary fat restriction and flaxseed supplementation in men with prostate cancer before surgery: exploring the effects on hormonal levels, prostate-specific antigen histopathologic features." *Urology.* 2001; 58 (1): 47-52.

Cameron, E. H. D., et al. "Benign and malignant breast disease in South Wales: a study of urinary steroids." *B MedJ.* 1990; 768-71.

Cameron, O. G., et al. "Venous plasma epinepherine levels and the symptoms of stress." *Psychosom Med.* 1990; 52 (4): 411-24.

Carette, S., et al. "Fibromyalgia and sex hormones." *J Rheumatol.* 1992; 9 (5): 831.

Carette, S., et al. "Fibrosis and primary hypothyroidism." *J Rheumatol.* 1988; 15: 1418-21.

Carlson, L.E., Sherwin, B.B. Steroid hormones, memory and mood in a healthy elderly population. *Psychoneuroendocrinology* 1998 Aug; 23(6): 583-603.

Caroff, S., et al. "Diurnal variation of growth hormone secretion following thyrotropin-releasing hormone infusion in normal men." *Psychosom Med.* 1989; 46 (1): 59.

Carroll, K. K., "Dietary fats and cancer." *Am J Clin Nutr.* 1991; 53: 1064S-67S.

Casson, P. R., et al. "Dehydroepiandrosterone supplementation augments ovarian stimulation in poor responders: a case series." *Hum Reprod.* 2000; 15 (10): 2129-32.

Chan, V., et al. "Urinary thyroxine excretion as an index of thyroid function." *Lancet.* 1972; 1 (7740): 4-6.

Chappel, M. R., "Infectious mononucleosis." *Southwest Med.* 1962; 43: 253-55.

Chen, F. P., et al. "Effects of hormone replacement therapy on cardiovascular risk factors in postmenopausal women." *Fertil Steril.* 1998; 69 (2): 267-73.

Chen, L. D., et al. "Melatonin's inhibitory effect on growth of ME-180 human cervical cancer cells is not related to intracellular glutathione concentrations." *Cancer Lett.* 1995; 91 (2): 153-59.

Cherrier, M. M., et al. "Testosterone supplementation improves spatial and verbal memory in healthy older men." *Neurology.* 2001; 57 (1): 80-88.

Chmouliovsky, L., et al. "Beneficial effect of hormone replacement therapy on weight loss in obese menopausal women." *Maturitas.* 1999; 32 (3): 147-53.

Chopra, I. J., et al. "Circulating thyroid hormones in thyrotropin in adult patients with proteincalorie malnutrition." *J Clin Endocrinol Metab.* 1975; 40: 221-27.

Choudhry, R., et al. "Localization of androgen receptors in human skin by immunohistochemistry: implications for the hormonal regulation of hair growth, sebaceous glands and sweat glands." *J Endocrinol.* 1992; 133 (3): 467-75.

Christiaansen, J. S., et al. "Kidney function and size in normal subjects before and during growth hormone administration for one week." *Ear J Clin Invest.* 1981; 11: 487-90.

Chuang, J. I., et al. "Melatonin decreases brain serotonin release, arterial pressure and heart rate in rats." *Pharmacology.* 1993; 47 (2): 91-97.

Chuang, J. I., et al. "Pharmacological effects of melatonin treatment on both locomotor activity and brain serotonin release in rats." *J Pineal Res.* 1994; 7 (1): 11-16.

Citera, G., et al. "The effect of melatonin in patients with fibromyalgia: a pilot study." *Clin Rheumatol.* 2000; 19 (1): 9-13.

Cittadini, A., et al. "Impaired cardiac performance in GH deficient adults and its improvement after GH replacement." *Am J Physiol.* 1994; 267 (2 Pt 1): E219-25.

Claustrat, B., et al. "Melatonin and jet lag: confirmatory result using a simplified protocol." *Biol Psychiatry.* 1992; 15; 32 (8): 705-11.

Cleare, A. J., et al. "Hypothalamo-pituitary-adrenal axis dysfunction in chronic fatigue syndrome the effects of low-dose hydrocortisone therapy." *J Clin Endocrinol Metab.* 2001; 86 (8): 3545-54.

Cleare, A. J., et al. "Urinary free cortisol in chronic fatigue syndrome." *Am J Psychiatry.* 2001; 158 (4): 641-43.

Cleghorn, R. A. "Adrenal cortisol insufficiency: psychological and neurological observations." *Canad Med Ass J.* 1951; 65: 449.

Clemmesen, B., et al. "Human growth hormone and growth hormone releasing hormone: a double-masked, placebo-controlled study of their effects on bone metabolism in elderly women." *Osteoporos Int.* 1993; 6: 330-36.

Coleman, D. L., et al. "Therapeutic effects of DHEA metabolites in diabetes mutant mice." *Endocrinology.* 1984; 115 (1): 239-43.

Collu, R., et al. "Role of catecholamines in the inhibitory effect of immobilisation stress on testosterone secretion in rats." *Biol. Reprod.* 1984; 30: 416-22.

Comstock, G. W., "The relationship of serum dehydroepiandrosterone and its sulfate to subsequent cancer of the prostate." *Cancer Epidemiol Biomarkers Prev.* 1993; 2 (3): 219-21.

Constant, E. L., et al. "Cerebral blood flow and glucose metabolism in hypothyroidism: a positron emission tomography study. " *J Clin Endocrinol Metab.* 2001; 86 (8): 3864-70.

Conti, E., et al. "Markedly reduced insulin-like growth factor-1 in the acute phase of myocardial infarction." *J Am Coll Cardiol.* 2001; 38 (1): 26-32.

Corpechot, C., et al. "Pregnenolone and its sulfate ester in the rat brain." *Brain Res.* 1983; 270 (1): 119-25.

Cos, S., et al. "Influence of melatonin on invasive and metastatic properties of MCF-7 human breast cancer cells." *Cancer Res.* 1998; 58 (19): 4383-90.

Cowan, L. D., et al. "Breast cancer incidence in women with a history of progesterone deficiency." *Am J Epidemiol.* 1981; 114 (2): 209-17.

Crane, M. G., et al. "Hypertension, oral contraceptive agents and conjugated estrogens." *Ann Intern Med.* 1971; 74: 13-21.

Crave, J. C., et al. "Effects of diet and metformin administration on sex hormone-binding globulin, androgens, and insulin in hirsute and obese women." *J Clin Endocrinol Metab.* 1995; 80 (7): 2057-62.

Criqui, M. H., et al. "Postmenopausal estrogen use and mortality: Results from a prospective study in a defined, homogeneous community." *Am J Epidemiol.* 1988;128:606-14.

Culebras, A., et al. "Differential response of growth hormone, cortisol, and prolactin to seizures and stress." *Epilepsie.* 1987; 28: 564-70.

Cuneo, R. C., et al. "Growth hormone treatment in growth hormone deficient adults. I. Effects on muscle mass and strength. " *J Appl Physiol.* 1991; 70 (2): 688-94.

Cuneo, R. C., et al. "Growth hormone treatment in growth hormone deficient adults. II. Effects on exercise performance." *J Appl Physiol.* 1991; 70 (2): 695-700.

Cuneo, R. C., et al. "Skeletal muscle performance in adults with growth hormone deficiency." *Horm Res.* 1990; 33 (Suppl 4): 55-60.

Currier, N. L., "Echinacea purpurea and melatonin augment natural-killer cells in leukemic mice and prolong life span."

Cutolo, M., et al. "The hypothalamic-pituitary-adrenocortical and gonadal axis function in rheumatoid arthritis." *Z Rheumatol.* 2000; 59 (Suppl 2): 11/65-69.

Dailey, M. P., et al. "Polymyalgia rheumatic begins at 40." *Arch Int Med.* 1979;139:743-74.

Darnaudery, M., et al. "The promnesic neurosteroid pregnenolone sulfate increases paradoxical sleep in rats." *Brain Res.* 1999; 818 (2): 492-98.

Davellaar, E. M., et al. "No increase in the incidence of breast carcinoma with subcutaneous administration of estradiol." *Ned Tijdsch Geneeskd.* 1991; 135 (14): 613-15.

Davis, S. R. "The clinical use of androgens in female sexual disorders. " *J Sex Marital Ther.* 1998; 24 (3): 153-63.

Davis, S. R., et al. "Effects of estradiol with and without testosterone on body composition and relationships with lipids in postmenopausal women." *Menopause.* 2000; 7 (6): 395-401.

De Peretti, E., et al. "Unconjugated dehydroepiandrosterone plasma levels in normal subjects from birth to adolescence in human: the use of a sensitive radioimmunoassay." *J Clin Endocrinol Metab.* 1976; 43 (5): 982-91.

De Pergola, G. "The adipose tissue metabolism: role of testosterone and dehydroepiandrosterone." *Int J Obes Relat Metab Disord.* 2000; 24 (Suppl 2): S59-63.

De Pergola, G., et al. "Body fat accumulation is possibly responsible for lower dehydroepiandrosterone circulating levels in premenopausal obese women." *Int J Obes Relat Metab Disord.* 1996; 20 (12): 1105-10.

De Pergola, G., et al. "Low dehydroepiandrosterone circulating levels in premenopausal obese women with very high body mass index." *Metabolism.* 1991; 40 (2): 187-90.

Degelau, J., et al. "The effect of DHEAs on influenza vaccination in aging adults." *J Am Geriatr Soc.* 1997; 45 (6): 747-51.

Degerblad, M., et al. "Physical and psychological capabilities during substitution therapy with recombinant growth hormone in adults with growth hormone deficiency." *Acta Endocrinol (Copenh).* 1990; 123: 185-93.

Deijen, J. B., et al. "Cognitive changes during growth hormone replacement in adult men." *Psychoneuroendocrinology.* 1998; 23 (1): 45-55.

Del Rio, G., et al. "Effect of estradiol on the sympathoadrenal response to mental stress in normal men." *J Clin Endocrinol Metab.* 1994; 79 (3): 836-40.

Delwaide, P. J., et al. "Acute effect of drugs upon memory of patients with senile dementia." *Acta Psychiatr Belg.* 1980; 80: 748-54.

Demitrack, M. A., et al. "Evidence for impaired activation of the hypothal-amic-pituitaryadrenal axis in patients with chronic fatigue syndrome." *J Clin Endocrinol Metab.* 1991; 73 (6): 1224-34.

Deplewski, D., et al. "Growth hormone and insulin-like growth factors have different effects on sebaceous cell growth and differentiation." *Endrocrinology.* 1999; 140 (9): 4089-94.

Dessein, P. H., et al. "Hyposecretion of adrenal androgens and the relation of serum adrenal steroids, serotonin and insulin-like growth factor-1 to clinical features in women with fibromyalgia." *Pain.* 1999; 83 (2): 313-19.

Dessein, P. H., et al. "Hyposecretion of the adrenal androgen dehydroepiandrosterone sulfate and its relation to clinical variables in inflammatory arthrosis." *Arthrosis Res.* 2001; 3 (3): 183-88.

Deutsch, S., et al. "The correlation of serum estrogens and androgens with bone density in the late postmenopause." *Int J Gynaecol Obstet.* 1987; 25 (3): 217-22.

Dhillon, V. B., et al. "Assessment of the effect of oral corticosteroids on bone mineral density in systemic lupus erythematosus: a preliminary study with dual energy x-ray absorptiometry." *Ann Rheum Dis.* 1990; 49 (8): 624-26.

Diallo, K., et al. "Inhibition of human immunodeficiency virus type-1 (HIV-1) replication by immunor (IM28), a new analog of dehydroepiandrosterone." *Nucleosides Nucleotides Nucleic Acids.* 2000; 19 (10-12): 2019-24.

Diamond. P., et al. "Metabolic effects of 12-month percutaneous dehydroepiandrosterone replacement therapy in postmenopausal women." *J Endocrinol.* 1996; 150 (Suppl): S43-50.

Dillman, E., et al. "Hypothermia in iron deficiency due to altered tri-iodothyronine metabolism.' *Am J Physiol.* 1980; 239: 377-81.

Dinan, T. G., et al. "Responses of growth hormone to desipramine in endogenous and Nonendogenous depression." *Br J Psychiatry.* 1990; 156: 680-84.

Dorgan, J. F., et al. "Effects of dietary fat and fiber on plasma and urine androgens and estrogens in men: a controlled feeding study." *Am J Clin Nutr.* 1996; 64 (6): 850-55.

Dorgan, J. F., et al. "Relation of energy, fat, and fiber intakes to plasma concentrations of estrogens and androgens in premenopausal women." *Am J Clin Nutr.* 1996; 64 (1): 2 5-31.

Dorwart, B. B., et al. "Joint effusions, chondrocalcinosis and other traumatic manifestations in hypothyroidism." *Am J Med.* 1975; 59: 780.

Dow, M. G., et al. "Hormonal treatments of sexual unresponsiveness in postmenopausal women: a comparative study." *Br J Obstet Gynaecol.* 1983; 90: 361-66.

Dubbels, R., et al. "Melatonin in edible plants identified by radioim-munoassay and by high performance liquid chromatography-mass spectrometry. " *J Pineal Res.* 1995; 18 (1): 28-31.

Ducceschi, V., et al. "Estrogens, left ventricular function and coronary circulation: what are the possibilities of therapeutic use?" *Minerva Cardioangiol.* 1995; 43 (4): 135-43.

Dudley, R. E., et al. "Comparative pharmacokinetics of three doses of percutaneous dihydrotestosterone gel in healthy elderly men – a clinical research center study." *J Clin Endocrinol Metab.* 1998; 83 (8): 2749-57.

Edwards, E. A., et al. "Testosterone propionate as a therapeutic agent in patients with organic disease of the peripheral vessels." *N Engl J Med.* 1939; 220: 865.

Elder, J., et al. "The relationship between serum cholesterol and serum thyrotropin, thyroxine and triiodothyronine concentrations in suspected hypothyroidism." *Ann Clin Biochem.* 1990; 27 (Pt 2): 110-13.

Eriksen, E. F., et al. "Growth hormone and insulin-like growth factors as anabolic therapies for osteoporosis." *Horm Res.* 1993; 40 (1-3): 95-98.

Erkkola, R. "Female menopause, hormone replacement therapy and cognitive processes." *Maturitas.* 1996; 23 suppl: 527-30.

Eschbach, J. W., et al. "Correction of the anemia of end-stage renal disease with recombinant human erythropoietin: results of a combined Phase I and II clinical trial." *N Engl J Med.* 1987; 316: 73-78.

Eulry, F., et al. "Bone density in differentiated cancer of the thyroid gland treated by hormone suppressive therapy." Study based on fifty-one cases. *Rev Rhum Mal Osteoartic.* 1992; 59 (4): 247-52.

Evans, W. S., et al. "Effects of in vivo gonadal hormone environment on in vitro hp GRF-40-stimulated GH release." *Am J Physiol.* 1985; 249: E276-80.

Everilt, A., et al. "Aging and anti-aging effects of hormones." *J Gerontol.* 1989: B139-47.

Everitt, A. V. In *Hypothalamus, pituitary and ageing.* Springfield, Illinois: Thomas; 68.

Fagard, R., "The role of exercise in blood pressure control: supportive evidence." *J Hypertension.* 1995; 13: 1223-27.

Fairfield, W. P., et al. "Effects of testosterone and exercise on muscle leanness in eugonadal men with AIDS wasting." *J Appl Physiol.* 2001; 90 (6):2166-71.

Falkheden, T., et al. "Renal function and kidney size following hypophysectomy in man." *Acta Endocrinol (Copenh).* 1965; 48: 348.

Fauci, A. S., "Immunosuppressive and anti-inflammatory effects of glucocorticoids." In Baxter, J. D., et al., eds. *Glucocorticoid Hormone Action.* New York: Springer-Verlag. 1979; 449-65.

Fava, M., et al. "Psychological behavioral and biochemical factors for coronary artery disease among American and Italian male corporate managers." *Am J Cardiol.* 1992; 70: 1412-16.

Fazekas, A. G., et al. "The metabolism of DHEA by human scalp hair follicles." *J Clin Endocrinol Metab.* 1973; 36: 582.

Feinhold, K. R., et al. "Endocrine-skin interactions. Cutaneous manifestations of pituitary disease, thyroid disease, calcium disorders and diabetes." *J Am Acad Dermatol.* 1987; 17 (6): 921-40.

Feldman, H. A., et al. "Low dehydroepiandrosterone and ischemic heart disease in middle-aged men: prospective results from the Masschusetts Male Aging Study." *Am J Epidemiol.* 2001; 153 (1): 79-89.

Ferrando, S. J., et al. "Dehydroepiandrosterone sulfate (DHEAs) and testosterone: relation to HIV illness stage and progression over one year." *J Acquir Immune Deft Syndr.* 1999; 22 (2): 146-54.

Fingerova, H., et al. "Reduced serum dehydroepiandrosterone levels in postmenopausal osteoporosis." *Ceska Gynekol.* 1998; 63 (2): 110-13.

Finkle, W. D., et al. "Endometrial cancer risk after discontinuing use of unopposed conjugated estrogens." *Cancer Causes Control.* 1995; 6 (2): 99-102.

Fish, I. R., et al. "Oral contraceptives and blood pressure." *J Am Med Assoc.* 1977;237:2499-503.

Fleming, M. W., et al. "Consequences of dose-dependent immunosuppression by progesterone on parasitic worm burdens in lambs." *Am J Vet Res.* 1993; 54 (8): 1299-302.

Flood, J. F. "DHEA and its sulfate enhance memory retention mice." *Brain Research.* 1988; 447: 269-78.

Flood, J. F. "Memory-enhancing effects in male mice of pregnenolone and steroids metabolically derived from it." *Proc Natl Acad Sci USA.* 1992; 89: 1567-71.

Flood, J. F., et al. "Age-related decrease of plasma testosterone in SAMP8 mice: replacement improves age-related impairment of learning and memory. *Physiol Behav.* 1995; 57 (4): 669-73.

Flood, J. F., et al. "Dehydroepiandrosterone sulfate improves memory in aging mice." *Brain Res.* 1988; 448 (1): 178-81.

Flood, J. F., et al. "Memory-enhancing effects in male mice of pregnenolone and steroids metabolically derived from it." *Proc Nail Acad Sci USA.* 1992; 89: 1567-71.

Foldes, J., et al. "Decreased serum IGF-I and dehydroepiandrosterone sulphate may be risk factors for the development of reduced bone mass in postmenopausal women with endogenous subclinical hyperthyroidism." *Eur J Endocrinol.* 1997; 136 (3): 277-81.

Fountoulakis, K. N., et al. "Morning and evening plasma melatonin and dexamethasone suppression test in patients with nonseasonal major depressive disorder from northern Greece (latitude 40-41.5 degrees)." *Neuropsychobiology.* 2001; 44 (3): 113-17.

Franklyn, J. A., et al. "Thyroxine replacement therapy and circulations rapid concentrations." *Clin Endocrinol (Oxf).* 1993; 38 (5): 453-59.

Fredrikson, M., et al. "Cortisol excretion during the defence reaction in humans." *Psychosom Med.* 1985; 47 (4): 313-19.

Freedman, D. S., et al. "Relation of serum testosterone levels to high density lipoprotein cholesterol and other characteristics in men." *Arterioscler Thromb.* 1991; (2): 307-15.

Freudenheim, J. L., et al. "Premenopausal breast cancer risk and intake of vegetables, fruits and related nutrients." *J Natl Cancer Inst.* 1996; 88: 340-48.

Friedl, K. E., et al. "Comparison of the effects of high dose testosterone and 19-nortestosterone to a replacement dose of testosterone on strength and body composition in normal men." *J Steroid Biochem Mol Biol.* 1991; 40 (4-6): 607-12.

Friedl, K. E., et al. "High-density lipoprotein cholesterol is not decreased if an aromatizable androgen is administered." *Metabolism.* 1990; 39 (1): 69-74.

Friedman, T. C., et al. "Decreased delta-sleep and plasma delta-sleepinducing peptide in patients with Cushing syndrome." *Neuroendocrinology.* 1994; 60 (6): 626-34.

Friedrich, M. "Effects of diet enrichment with glucose and casein on blood cortisol concentration of calves in early postnatal period." *Arch Vet Pol.* 1995; 35 (1-2): 117-25.

Friess, E., et al. "DHEA administration increases rapid eye movement sleep and EEG power in the sigma frequency range." *Am Physiological Society.* 1995; E107-13.

Frohlich, M., et al. "Effects of hormone replacement therapies on fibrinogen and plasma viscosity in postmenopausal women." *Br J Haematol.* 1998; 100 (3): 577-81.

Fuller, H. Jr., et al. "Myxedema and hypertension." *Postgrad. Med.* 1966; 40: 425-28.

Furman, R. H., et al. "Effect of androgens and estrogens on serum lipids and the composition and concentration of serum lipoproteins in normolipemic and hyperlipidemic states." *Proc Biochem Pharmacol.* 1967; 12: 215-49.

Fuyns, A., "Alcohol and cancer." *Proc Nutr Soc.* 1990; 49: 145-51.

Gaillard, R. C., et al. "Stress and pituitary adrenal axis." *Bailliere's Clin End Metab.* 1987; 1 (2): 319-54.

Gambrell, R. D., Jr. "Hormones in the etiology and prevention of breast and endometrial cancer." *South Med J.* 1984; 77 (12): 1509-15.

Gambrell, R. D., Jr., et al. "Decreased incidence of breast cancer in post-menopausal estrogenprogestogen users." *Obstet Gynecol.* 1983; 62 (4): 435-43.

Garfinkel, D., et al. "Improvement of sleep quality in elderly people by controlled-release melatonin." *Lancet.* 1995; 346 (8974): 541-44.

Garnero, P., et al. "Biochemical markers of bone turnover, endogenous hormones and the risk of fractures in postmenopausal women: the OFELY study." *J Bone Miner Res.* 2000; 15 (8): 1526-36.

Garro, A., et al. "Alcohol and Cancer." *Ann Rev Pharmacol Toxicol.* 1990; 30: 219-49.

Gauchie, C., et al. "The relationship between testosterone levels and cognition ability patterns." *Psychoneuroendocrinology.* 1991; 16 (4): 323-34.

Gerhard, M., et al. "Estradiol therapy combined with progesterone and endothelium-dependent vasodilation in postmenopausal women." *Circulation.* 1998; 98 (12): 1158-63.

Geyelin, H. R., et al. *J Metab Res.* 1922; 767-91.

Giagulli, V. A., et al. "Pathogenesis of the decreased androgen levels in obese men. *J Clin Endocrinol Metab.* 1994; 79 (4): 997-1000.

Giltay, E. J., et al. "Effects of sex steroid deprivation/administration on hair growth and skin sebum production in transsexual males and females." *J Clin Endocrinol Metab.* 2000; 85 (8): 2913-21.

Ginsburg, E. "Effects of alcohol ingestion on estrogens in postmenopausal women." *JAMA.* 1996; 276 (21): 1747-51.

Golding, D. N., "Hypothyroidism presenting with musculo-skeletal symptoms." *Ann Rheum Dis.* 1970; 29: 10-14.

Golditz, G. A., et al. "Increased green and yellow vegetable intake and lowered cancer deaths in an elderly population." *Am J Clin Nutr.* 1985; 41 (1): 326.

Goldman, R, Klatz, R . Stopping the Clock- 1996.

Gordon, G. B. "Relationship of serum levels of DHEA and DHEAs to the risk of developing postmenopausal breast cancer." *Cancer Res.* 1990; 50: 3859-62.

Gordon, G. B., "Reduction of atherosclerosis by administration of DHEA." *J Clin. Invest.* 1988; 82: 712-20.

Gordon, T., et al. "Drinking and coronary heart disease: the Albary study." *Am Heart J.* 1985; 110: 331-34.

Gower, D. B., et al. "Comparison of 16-androstene steroid concentrations in sterile apocrine sweat and axillary secretions: interconversions of 16-androstenes by the axillary microflora – a mechanism for axillary odour production in man." *J Steroid Biochem Mol Biol* 1994; 48 (4): 409-18.

Grad, B. R., et al. "The role of melatonin and serotonin in aging: update." Published erratum appears in *Psychoneuroendocrinology.* 1993; 18 (7): 541.

Granner, D. K. "The role of glucocorticoid hormones as biologic amplifiers." In *Glucocorticoid Hormone Action,* Baxter, J. D., et al., eds. New York: Springer-Verlag, 1979; 593-611.

Greenblatt, R.B., Oettinger, M., Bohler, C.S. Estrogen-androgen levels in aging men and women: therapeutic considerations. *J. Am. Geriatr. Soc.* 1976 Apr; 24(4): 173-8.

Grinspoon, S., et al. "Body composition and endocrine function in women with acquired immunodeficiency syndrome wasting." *J Clin Endocrinol Metab.* 1997; 82 (5): 1332-37.

Grinspoon, S., et al. "Effect of androgen administration in men with the AIDS wasting syndrome. A randomized, double-blind, placebo-controlled trial." *Ann Intern Med.* 1998; 129 (1): 18-26.

Grinspoon, S., et al. "Loss of lean body and muscle mass correlates with androgen levels in hypogonadal men with acquired immunodeficiency syndrome and wasting." *J Clin Endocrinol Metab.* 1996; 8 (11): 4051-58.

Grodstein, F., et al. "A prospective, observational study of postmenopausal hormone therapy and primary prevention of cardiovascular disease." *Ann Intern Med.* 2000; 133 (12): 933-41.

Gros, H. A., et al. "Effect of biologically active steroids on thyroid function in man" *J Clin Endocrinol Metab.* 1975; 33: 242.

Grunfeld, C., et al. "Indices of thyroid function and weight loss in human immunodeficiency virus infection and the acquired immunodeficiency syndrome." *Metabolism.* 1993; 42 (10): 1270-76.

Guay, A. T. "Decreased testosterone in regularly menstruating women with decreased libido: a clinical observation." *J Sex Marital Ther.* 2001; 27 (5): 513-19.

Gumbatov, N. B., et al. "State of the hypophyseal-gonadal system in patients with hypertension during long-term treatment with nadolol and anaprilin." *Kardiologia.* 1991; 31 (4): 15-18.

Gutai, J., et al. "Plasma testosterone, high density lipoprotein cholesterol and other lipoprotein factions." *Am J Cardiol.* 1981; 48: 897-902.

Hadley, O., et al. "Adrenal androgens and cortisol in major depression." *Am J Psychiatry.* 1993; 150 (5): 806-9.

Halpern, C. T., et al. "Monthly measures of salivary testosterone predict sexual activity in adolescent males." *Arch Sex Behav.* 1998; 27 (5): 445-65.

Hamilton, J. B., "Increased levels of circulating testosterone can cause scalp hair loss in susceptible individuals." *Amer J Anat.* 1992; 71: 451.

Hammond, C. B., et al. "Current status of estrogen therapy for the menopause." *Fertil Steril.* 1982; 37: 5-25.

Hanke, H., et al. "Estradiol concentrations in premenopausal women with coronary heart disease." *Coron Artery Dis.* 1997; 8 (8-9): 511-15.

Harro, J., et al. "Association of depressiveness with blunted growth hormone response to maximal physical exercise in young healthy men." *Psychoneuroendocrinology.* 1999; 24 (5): 505-17.

Hassager, C., et al. "Collagen synthesis in postmenopausal women during therapy with anabolic steroid or female sex hormones." *Metabolism.* 1990; 39 (11): 1167-69.

Hassager, C., et al. "Estrogen/proestagen therapy changes soft tissue body composition in postmenopausal women." *Metabolism.* 1989; 38 (7): 662-65.

Hattori, A., et al. "Identification of melatonin in plants and its effects on plasma melatonin levels and binding to melatonin receptors in vertebrates." *Biochem Mol Biol Int.* 1995; 35 (3): 627-34.

Hayashi, T., et al. "Dehydroepiandrosterone retards atherosclerosis formation through its conversion to estrogen: the possible role of nitric oxide." *Arte-rioscler Thromb Vasc Biol.* 2000; 20 (3): 782-92.

Healey, L. A., "Polymyalgia rheumatica." In Hollander, J. L., et al., eds. *Arthritis and Allied Conditions,* 8th ed., Philadelphia: Lea and Febiger, 1972; 885-89.

Heikkila, R., et al. "Serum androgen-anabolic hormones and the risk of rheumatoid arthritis." *Ann Rheum Dis.* 1998; 57 (5): 281-85.

Henderson, E., et al. "Pregnenolone." *J Clin Endocrinol.* 1950; 10: 455-74.

Herrington D. "DHEA and atherosclerosis." *Ann NY Acad Sci.* 1999; 774: 271-80.

Herrington, O., et al. "Plasma DHEA and DHEAs in patients undergoing diagnostic coronary angiography." *J Am Coll Cardiol.* 1990; 16: 862-70.

Herrinton, L. J., et al. "Postmenopausal unopposed estrogens. Characteristics of use in relation to the risk of endometrial carcinoma." *Ann Epidemiol.* 1993; 3 (3): 308-18.

Hertoghe, T., "Growth hormone therapy in aging adults." In Anti-Aging Medical Therapeutics, R. M. Klatz. et al., eds. Marina Del Rey, California: *Health Quest Publications,* 1997; 10-28.

Hertoghe, T., "The beneficial effects of hormone replacement therapies on obesity." *Anti-Aging Medical Therapeutics.* eds. R. M. Klatz and B. Goldman. Marina Del Rey, California: Health Quest Publications, 2001.

Hertoghe, T., "Thyroid Diagnosis and Treatment. Many conditions related to age reduce the conversion of thyroxine to triiodothyronine, a rationale for prescribing preferentially a combined T3 + T4 preparation in hypothyroid adults." Anti-Aging Medical therapeutics; eds. R. M. Klatz and B. Goldman. Marina Del Rey, California: Health Quest Publications, 2000; 138-53.

Hertoghe, T., "The Hormone Solution- Staying Younger Longer with Natural Hormones and Nutritional Therapies" 2002

Hertoghe, T., "Thyroid Diagnosis and Treatment. Poor reliability of the single plasma TSH-test for diagnosis of thyroid dysfunction and follow-up." Anti-Aging Medical Therapeutics, eds. R. M. Klatz and B. Goldman- Marina Del Rey, California: Health Quest Publications, 2000; 127-37.

Hertoghe, T., et al. "Considerable improvement of hypothyroid symptoms with two combined T3-T4 medication in patients still symptomatic with thyroxine treatment alone." In press.

Herxheimer, A., "Melatonin for preventing and treating jet lag." *Cochrane Database Syst Rev.* 2001; 1: CD001520.

Heymann, W., "Cutaneous manifestations of thyroid disease." *J Am Acad Dermatol.* 1992; 26: 885-902.

Hill, P. B., et al. "Effect of a vegetarian diet and dexamethasone on plasma prolactin, testosterone and dehydroepiandrosterone in men and women." *Cancer Lett.* 1979; 7 (5): 273-82.

Hill, S. R., Jr., et al. "The role of the endocrine glands in the rheumatic diseases." In Hollander, J. L. ed. *Arthritis and Allied Conditions,* 7th ed., Philadelphia: Lea & Febiger, 1966; 597-605.

Hollander, L. E., et al. "Sleep quality, estradiol levels, and behavioral factors in late reproductive age women." *Obstet Gynecol.* 2001; 98 (3): 391-97.

Holmdahl, R., et al. "Oestrogen is a potent immunomodulator of murine experimental rheumatoid arthritis." *Br J Rheum,* 1989; 28 (suppl 1): 54.

Holmes, S. J., et al. "Reduced bone mineral density in patients with adult onset growth hormone deficiency." *J Clin Endocrinol Metab.* 1994; 78 (3): 669-74.

Hromadova, M., et al. "Alterations of lipid metabolism in men with hypotestosteronemia." *Horm Metab Res.* 1991; 23 (8): 392-94.

Hughes, G. S., et al. "Fish oil produces an atherogenic lipid profile in hypertensive men."

Atherosclerosis. 1990; 84 (2-3): 229-37.

Hulley, S., et al. "Randomized trial of estrogen plus progestin for secondary prevention of coronary heart disease in postmenopausal women. Heart and Estrogen/progestin Replacement Study (HERS) Research Group." *JAMA.* 1998; 280 (7): 605-13.

Hunt, P. J., et al. "Improvement in mood and fatigue after dehy-droepiandrosterone replacement in Addison's disease in a randomized, double-blind trial." *J Clin Endocrinol Metab.* 2000; 85 (12): 4650-56.

Imperato-McGinley, J. J., et al. "The androgen control of sebum production. Studies of subjects with dihydrotestosterone deficiency and complete androgen insensitivity." *J Clin Endocrinol Metab.* 1993; 76: 524-28.

Inagaki, N., et al. "Drugs for the treatment of allergic diseases." *Jpn J Pharmacol.* 2001; 86 (3): 275-80. Review.

Ingram, D. M., et al. "Effect of low-fat diet on female sex hormone levels." *J Natl Cancer Inst.* 1987; 79 (6): 1225-29.

Inoh, H., et al. "Correlation between the age of pinealectomy and the development of scoliosis in chickens." *Spine.* 2001; 26 (9): 1014-21.

Iranmanesh, A., et al. "Age and relative adiposity are specific negative determinants of the frequency and amplitude of growth hormone (GH) secretory bursts and the half-life of endogenous GH in healthy men." *J Clin Endocrinol Metab.* 1991; 73 (5): 1081-88.

Israel, N., "An effective therapeutic approach to atherosclerosis illustrating harmlessness of prolonged use of thyroid hormone in coronary disease." *Am J Dig Dis.* 1955; 22: 161-68.

Iversen, P., et al. "Serum testosterone as a prognostic factor in patients with advanced prostatic carcinoma." *Scand J Urol Nephrol Suppl.* 1994; 157: 41-47.

Jacubinovicz, D., et al. "Disparate effects of weight reduction by diet on serum DHEA in obese men and women. " *J Clin Endocrinol Metab.* 1993; 80 (11) 3373-76.

Jansson, J. H., et al. "Von Willebrand factor, tissue plasminogen activator, and dehydroepiandrosterone sulphate predict cardiovascular death in a 10-year follow-up of survivors of acute myocardial infarction." *Heart.* 1998; 80 (4): 334-37.

Jarett, D. B., et al. "Sleep-related growth hormone secretion is persistently suppressed in women with recurrent depression: a preliminary longitudinal analysis." *J Psychiatr Res.* 1994; 28 (3): 211-23.

Jean-Louis, G., et al. "Melatonin effects on sleep, mood, and cognition in elderly with mild cognitive impairment." *J Pineal Res.* 1998; 25 (3): 177-83.

Jick, S. S., et al. "Estrogens, progesterone, and endometrial cancer." *Epidemiology.* 1993; 4 (1): 20-24.

Johannes, C. B., et al. "Relation of dehydroepiandrosterone and dehydroepiandrosterone sulfate with cardiovascular disease risk factors in women: longitudinal results from the Massachusetts Women's Health Study." *J Clin Epidemiol.* 1999; 52 (2): 95-103.

Johansson, G., et al. "Examination stress affects plasma levels of TSH and thyroid hormone differently in females and males." *Psychosom Med.* 1987; 49: 390-96.

Jolin, T., et al. "The different effects of thyroidectomy, KCIO4, and propyl-thiouracil on insulin secretion and glucose uptake in the rat." *Endocrinology.* 1974; 94: 1502.

Jungmann, E., et al. "Somatomedin C level and stimulation of growth hormone and adrenal cortex function by administration of releasing hormones and physical exertion in patients with obesity." *Med Klin.* 1991; 86 (5): 237-40.

Kalk, W J., et al. "Thyroid hormone and carrier protein interrelationships in children recovering from kwashiorkor." *Am J Clin Nutr.* 1986; 43 (3): 406-13.

Kampen, D. L., et al. "Estradiol is related to visual memory in healthy young men." *Behav Neurosci.* 1996; 110 (3): 613-17.

Kapitola, J., "Hemodynamic effects of dehydroepiandrosterone in rats." *Agressologie.* 1972; 13 (4): 247-51.

Karasek, M., et al. "Pineal gland, melatonin and cancer." *Neuroendocrinol Lett.* 1999; 20 (3-4): 139-44.

Kass, E. H., et al. "Corticosteroids and infections." *Afr Intern Med.* 1958; 9: 45-80.

Kayumov, L., et al. "A randomized, double-blind, placebo-controlled crossover study of the effect of exogenous melatonin on delayed sleep phase syndrome." *Psychosom Med.* 2001; 63 (1): 40-48.

Keagy, E. M., et al. "Thyroid function, energy balance, body composition and organ growth in protein-deficient chicks." *J Nutr.* 1987; 117 (9): 1532-40.

Keast, Jr., et al. "Testosterone has potent, selective effects on the morphology of pelvic autonomic neurons which control the bladder, lower bowel and internal reproductive organs of the male rat." *Neuroscience.* 1998; 85 (2): 543-56.

Keefe, D. L., et al. "Hormone replacement therapy may alleviate sleep apnea in menopausal women: a pilot study." *Menopause.* 1999; 6 (3): 196-200.

Kelly, W. K., et al. "Prospective evaluation of hydrocortisone and suramin in patients with androgen-independent prostate cancer." *J Clin Oncol.* 1995; 13 (9): 2208-13.

Kenny, A. M., et al. "Effects of transdermal testosterone on bone and muscle in older men with low bioavailable testosterone levels." *J Gerontol A Biol Sci Med Sci.* 2001; 56 (5): M266-72.

Khorram, O., et al. "Activation of immune function by dehydroepiandrosterone (DHEA) in age-advanced men." *J Gerontol A Biol Sci Med Sci.* 1997; 52 (1): M1-7.

Kinson, G. A., et al. "Influences of anabolic androgens on cardiac growth and metabolism in the rat." *Can J Physiol Pharmacol.* 1991; 69 (11): 1698-704.

Knussmann, R., et al. "Relationship between sex hormones level and characters of hair and skin in healthy young men." *Am J Phys Anthropol.* 1992; 88 (1): 59-67.

Kopp, C. B., et al. "Relationship between sex hormones and haemostatic factors in healthy middle-aged men." *Atherosclerosis.* 1988; 71: 71-76.

Koppeschaar, H. P., "Growth hormone, insulin-like growth factor I and cognitive function in adults." *Growth Horm IGF Res.* 2000; 10 Suppl B: S69-73.

Kornhauser, C., et al. "The effect of hormone replacement therapy on blood pressure and cardiovascular risk factors in menopausal women with moderate hypertension." *J Hum Hypertens.* 1997; 11 (7): 405-11.

Krane, S. M., et al. "The skeletal system." Ingbar, S., et al., eds. In *Werner's the Thyroid.* Philadelphia: Lippincott Company, 1986; 1205.

Krentz, A. J., et al. "Anthropometric, metabolic, and immunological effects of recombinant human growth hormone in AIDS and AIDS-related complex." *J Acquir Immune Defic Syndr.* 1993; 6 (3): 245-51.

Krieg, M., et al. "Demonstration of a specific androgen receptor in rat heart muscle: relationship between binding, metabolism, and tissue levels of androgens." *Endocrinology.* 1978; 1686-94.

Kritz-Silverstein, D., et al. "Long-term postmenopausal hormone use, obesity and fat distribution in older women." *J AMA.* 1996; 276 (1).

Labrie, F., et al. "Effect of 12-month dehydroepiandrosterone replacement therapy on bone, vagina, and endometrium in postmenopausal women." *J Clin Endocrinol Metab.* 1997; 82 (10): 3498-505.

Laffargue, F., et al. "Estrogens, progestins and cancer of the endometrium." *Rev Prat.* 1993; 43 (20): 2603-9.

Lammoglia, M. A., et al. "Effects of dietary fat on follicular development and circulating concentrations of lipids, insulin, progesterone, estradiol-17 beta,13, 14-dihydro-15-ketoprostaglandin F(2 alpha) GH in estrous cyclic Brahman cows." *J Anim Sci.* 1997; 75 (6): 1591-600.

Landin-Wilhelmsen, K., et al. "Serum insulin-like growth factor in a random population sample of men and women: relation to age, sex, smoking habits, coffee consumption and physical activity, blood pressure and concentrations of plasma lipids, fibrinogen, parathyroid hormone and osteocalkin." *Clin Endocrinol (Oxf).* 1994; 41 (3): 351-57.

Langer, M., et al. "Androgen receptors, serum androgen levels and survival of breast cancer patients." *Arch Gynecol Obstet.* 1990; 247 (4): 203-9.

Lanthier, A., et al. "Sex steroids and 5-en-3 beta-hydroxysteroids in specific regions of the human brain and cranial nerves." *J Steroid Biochem.* 1986; 25: 445-49.

Laragh, J. H., "Oral contraceptive-induced hypertension. Nine years later." *Am J Obstet Gynecol.* 1976; 126: 141-47.

Lau, E. M., et al. "Risk factors for hip fracture in Asian men and women: the Asian osteoporosis study." *J Bone Miner Res.* 2001; 16 (3): 572-80.

Lauritzen, C., et al. "Risks of endometrial and mammary cancer morbidity and mortality in longterm estrogen treatment." In van Herendael, H., et al. *The Climacteric – An Update.* Lancaster, England: MTP Press Ltd, 1984; 207.

Leedy, M. G., et al. "Testosterone and cortisol levels in crewmen of U. S. air force fighter and cargo planes." *Psychosom Med.* 1985; 47 (4): 333-38.

Leenen, R., et al. "Visceral fat accumulation in relation to sex hormones in obese men and women undergoing weight loss therapy. "*J Clin Endocrinol Metab.* 1994; 78(6): 1515-20.

Li Voon Chong, J. S., et al. "Elderly people with hypothalamic-pituitary disease and growth hormone deficiency: lipid profiles, body composition and quality of life compared with control subjects." *Clin Endocrinol (Oxf).* 2000; 53 .(5): 551-59.

Lieberman, J. A., et al. "Acute antidepressant effect of lithium in unipolar depression." *Psychosomatics.* 1984; 25 (12): 932-33.

Lieberman, S. A., et al. "Anabolic effects of recombinant insulin-like growth factor." in cachectic patients with the acquired immunodeficiency syndrome. "*J Clin Endocrinol Metab.* 1994; 78 (2): 404-10.

Lieberman HR, Waldhauser F, Garfield G, et al. Effects of melatonin on human mood and performance. Brain Res (Netherlands) 323(2): 201-7, 1984.

Liechty, R. D., et al. "Cancer and thyroid function." *JAMA.* 1963; 183 (1): 116-18.

Linkowski, P., et al. "24-hour profiles of adrenocorticotropin, cortisol growth hormone in major depressive illness: effect of antidepressant treatment." *J Clin Endocrinol Metab.* 1987; 65 (1): 141-52.

Lissoni, P., et al. "Modulation of cancer endocrine therapy by melatonin: a phase II study of tamoxifen plus melatonin in metastatic breast cancer patients progressing under tamoxifen alone." *Br J Cancer.* 1995; 71 (4): 854-56.

Lomo, P. O., et al. "Respiratory activity of isolated liver Mitochondria following Trypanosoma congolense infection in rabbits: the role of thyroxine." *Com Biochem Physiol B.* 1993; 104 (1):187-91.

Lundgren, S., et al. "Influence of progestins on serum hormone levels in postmenopausal women with advanced breast cancer -II. A differential effect of megestrol acetate and medroxyprogesterone acetate on serum estrone sulfate and sex hormone binding globulin." *J Steroid Biochem.* 1990; 36 (1-2): 105-9.

Luo, S., et al. "Combined effects of dehydroepiandrosterone and EM-800 on bone mass, serum lipids the development of dimethylbenz(A)anthracene-induced mammary carcinoma in the rat." *Endocrinology.* 1997; 138 (10): 4435-44.

Lurie, M. B., et al. "On the role of the thyroid in native resistance to tuberculosis I. Effect of hyperthyroidism. II. Effect of hypothyroidism. The mode of action of thyroid hormones." *Am Rev Tuberc.* 1959; 79: 152-203.

Ly, L. P., et al. "A double-blind, placebo-controlled, randomized clinical trial of transdermal dihydrotestosterone gel on muscular strength, mobility quality of life in older men with partial androgen deficiency." *J Clin Endocrinol Metab.* 2001; 86 (9): 4078-88.

Maestroni, G. J. "Therapeutic potential of melatonin in immunodeficiency states, viral diseases cancer." *Adv Exp Med Biol.* 1999; 467: 2 17-26.

Maestroni, G. J., "The immunotherapeutic potential of melatonin." *Expert Opin Investig Drugs.* 2001; 10 (3): 467-76.

Maestroni, G. J., "Therapeutic potential of melatonin in immunodeficiency states, viral diseases cancer." *Adv Exp Med Biol.* 1999; 467: 217-26.

Maghnie, M., et al. "Diagnosing GH deficiency: the value of short-term hypocaloric diet." *J Clin Endocrinol Metab.* 1983; 77 (5): 1372-78.

Mann, D. R., et al. "Preservation of bone mass in hypogonadal female monkeys with recombinant human growth hormone administration." *J Clin Endocrinol Metab.* 1992; 74 (6): 1263-69.

Manson JE., Postmenopausal hormone replacement and atherosclerotic disease. *American Heart Journal.* 1994;128:1337-1343.

Marcus, M. A; et al. "Insulin sensitivity and serum triglyceride level in obese white and black women: relationship to visceral and truncal subcutaneous fat." *Metabolism.* 1999; 48 (2): 194-99.

Marek, J. "The significance of ovarian and testicular steroids in lipid metabolism and atherogenesis." *Vnitr Lek.* 1992; 38 (9): 913-20.

Marin, P., "Metabolic and gastrointestinal drugs: testosterone and regional fat distribution." *Obesity Res.* 1995; 3 (suppl 4): 6095-125.

Marin, P., et al. "Cortisol secretion in relation to body fat distribution in obese premenopausal women." *Metabolism.* 1992; 41 (8): 882-86.

Martens, H. F., et al. "Decreased testosterone levels in men with rheumatoid arthritis: effect of low dose prednisone therapy." *J Rheumatol.* 1994; 21 (8): 1427-31.

Mateiko, G. B., et al. "The efficacy of the hormonal substitute therapy of adolescents with viral hepatitis A combined with thyroid hypofunction." *Vrach Delo.* 1990; (8): 101-2.

Mathur, P. P., et al. "Effect of sleep deprivation on the physiological status of rat testis." *Andrologia.* 1991; 23 (1): 49-51.

Matteo, L., et al. "Sex hormones status and bone mineral density in men with rheumatoid arthritis." *J Rheumatol.* 1995; 22 (8): 1455-60.

Mayo, W., et al. "Pregnenolone sulfate and aging of cognitive functions: behavioral, neurochemical morphological investigations." *Horm Behav.* 2001; 40 (2): 215-17.

McCaul, K. D., et al. "Winning, losing, mood testosterone." *Horm Behav.* 1992; 26 (4): 486-504.

McCormick, D. L., et al. "Chemoprevention of hormone-dependent prostate cancer in the Wistar-Unilever rat." *Eur Urol.* 1999; 35 (5-6): 464-67.

McCormick, D. L., et al. "Exceptional chemopreventive activity of low-dose dehydroepiandrosterone in the rat mammary gland." *Cancer Res.* 1996; 56 (8): 1724-26.

McGauley, G. A., et al. "Psychological well-being before and after growth hormone treatment in adults with growth hormone deficiency." *Horm Res.* 1990; 33 (Suppl 4): 52-54.

McGavack, T., et al. "The use of pregnenolone in various clinical disorders." *J Clin Endocrinol.* 1951; 11: 559-77.

Melchior, C. L., et al. "Dehydroepiandrosterone is an anxiolytic in mice on the plus maze." *Pharmacol Biochem Behav.* 1994; 47 (3): 437-41.

Mellemgaard, A., et al. "Cancer risk in individuals with benign thyroid disorders." *Thyroid.* 1998; 8 (9): 751-54.

Mendenhall, C. L., et al. "Anabolic steroid effects on immune function: differences between analogues." *J Steroid Biochem Mol Biol.* 1990; 37 (1): 71-76.

Menof, P., "New method for control of hypertension." *S Afr Med J.* 1950; 24: 172.

Messina, M., et al. "The role of soy products in reducing the risk of cancer." *J Natl Cancer Inst.* 1991; 83: 541-46.

Meston, C. M., et al. "The neurobiology of sexual function." *Arch Gen Psychiatry.* 2000; 57 (11): 1012-30.

Meyer, N. A., et al. "Combined IGF-1 and growth hormone improves weight loss and wound healing in burned rats." *J Trauma.* 1996; 1 (6): 1008-12.

Meyerhoff, J. L., et al. "Psychologic stress increases plasma levels of prolactin, cortisol and POMC-derived peptides in man." *Psychosom Med.* 1988; 50: 28-29.

Miell, J. P., et al. "Effects of hypothyroidism and hyperthyroidism on insulin-like growth factors (IGFs) and growth hormone- and IGF-binding proteins." *J Clin Endocrinol Metab.* 1993; 76: 950-55.

Miller, L. H., et al. "A neuroheptapeptide influence on cognitive functioning in the elderly." *Peptides.* 1980; 55-57.

Mills, T. M., et al. "Androgens and penile erection: a review." *J Androl.* 1996; 17 (6): 633-38.

Minshall, R. D., et al. "Ovarian steroid protection against coronary artery hyperactivity in Rhesus Monkey." *J Clin Endocrinol Metab.* 1988; 83: 649-59.

Mishra, K. K., et al. "A study on physiological changes in essential hypertension and rheumatoid arthritis with reference to the levels of cortisol, blood glucose, triglycerides and cholesterol." *Indian J Physiol Pharmacol.* 1995; 39 (1): 68-70.

Mohan, P. F., et al. "Effects of DHEA treatment in rats with diet-induced obesity." *Nutrition Pharmacology & Toxicology.* 1990: 1103-14.

Montagna W, et al., eds. *The biology of hair growth.* New York: Academic Press, 1958; 355.

Mollefi, J., et al. "Effects of growth hormone administration on fuel oxidation and thyroid function in normal man." *Metabolism.* 1992; 41: 728.

Molsa, P. K., et al. "Epidemiology of dementia in a Finnish population." *Acta Neurol Scand.* 1982; 654: S41-S52.

Monroe, R. T., "Chronic arthritis in hyperthyroidism and myxedema." *N Engl J Med* 1935; 121: 1074.

Montgomery, B. M., et al. "Effect of oestrogen and testosterone implants on psychological disorders in the climacteric." *Lancet.* 1987; 1 (8528): 297-99.

Monti, J. M., et al. "A critical assessment of the melatonin effect on sleep in humans." *Biol Signals Recept.* 2000; 9 (6): 328-39.

Montplaisir, J., et al. "Sleep in menopause: differential effects of two forms of hormone replacement therapy." *Menopause.* 2001; 8 (1): 10-16.

Moorkens, G., et al. "Characterization of pituitary function with emphasis on GH secretion in the chronic fatigue syndrome." *Clin Endocrinol (Oxf).* 2000; 53 (1): 99-106.

Morabia, A., et al. "Thyroid hormones and duration of ovulatory activity in the etiology of breast cancer." *Cancer Epidemiol Biomakers Prev.* 1992; 1 (5): 389-93.

Morales, A., et al. "Androgen therapy in advanced carcinoma of the prostate." *CMA Journal.* 1971; 105: 71-72.

Morales, A., et al. "Effects of replacement dose of DHEA in men and women of advancing age." *J Clin Endocrinol Metab.* 1994; 78: 1360-67.

Mortola, J. F., et al. "The effect of oral DHEA on endocrine-metabolic parameters in postmenopausal women." *J Clin Endocrinol Metab.* 1990; 71 (3): 696-704.

Mortola, J. F., et al. "The effects of oral dehydroepiandrosterone on endocrine-metabolic parameters in postmenopausal women." *J Clin Endocrinol Metab.* 1990; 71 (3): 696-704.

Mullin, G. E., et al. "Cutaneous signs of thyroid disease." *Am Fam Physician.* 1989; 34 (4): 93-98.

Munzer, T., et al. "Effects of GH and/or sex steroid administration on abdominal subcutaneous and visceral fat in healthy aged women and men." *J Clin Endocrinol Metab.* 2001; 86 (8): 3604-10.

Murialdo, G., et al. "Circadian secretion of melatonin and thyrotropin in hospitalized aged patients." *Aging (Milano).* 1993; 5 (1): 39-46.

Möller, J. *Cholesterol: interactions with testosterone and cortisol in cardiovascular diseases.* Berlin Heidelberg: Springer-Verlag, 1987.

Nachtigall, L. E., et al. "Estrogen replacement II: A prospective study in the relationship to carcinoma and cardiovascular and metabolic problems." *Obstet Gynecol.* 1979; 54: 74.

Nagant de Deuxchaisnes, C., et al. "New modes of administration of salmon calcitonin in Paget's disease." *Clin Orthop Rel Res.* 1987; 217: 56-7 1.

Nagata, C., et al. "Association of dehydroepiandrosterone sulfate with serum HDL-cholesterol concentrations in post-menopausal Japanese women." *Maturitas.* 1998; 31 (1): 21-27.

Nagata, C., et al. "Serum concentrations of estradiol and dehydroepiandrosterone sulfate and soy product intake in relation to psychologic well-being in peri- and postmenopausal Japanese women." *Metabolism.* 2000; 49 (12): 1561-64.

Nave, R., et al. "Melatonin improves evening napping." *Eur J Pharmacol.* 1995; 275 (2): 213-16.

Neidel, J., "Changes in systemic levels of insulin-like growth factors and their binding proteins in patients with rheumatoid arthritis." *Clin Exp Rheumatol.* 2001; 19 (1): 81-84.

Nestler, J. E., et al. "DHEA reduces serum low density lipoprotein levels and body fat but does not alter insulin sensitivity in normal men." *J Clin Endocrinol Metab.* 1988; 66(1): 57-61.

Nicoloff, J. T, et al. "Altered peripheral thyroxine metabolism in severe obesity." *Clin Res.* 1966; 14: 148.

Niepomniszcze, H., et al. "Skin disorders and thyroid diseases." *J Endocrinol Invest.* 2001; 24 (8): 628-38.

Niskonen, L., et al. "The effects of weight loss on insulin sensitivity, skeletal muscle composition and capillary density in obese non-diabetic subjects." *Int J Obes Relat Metab Disord.* 1996; 20 (2): 154-60.

Noble, D. E., et al. "Localization of the growth hormone receptor/binding protein in skin." *Endocrinol.* 1990; 126 (3): 467-71.

Norton, S. D., et al. "Administration of dehydroepiandrosterone sulfate retards onset but not progression of autoimmune disease in NZB/W mice." *Autoimmunity.* 1997; 26 (3): 161-71.

Nowata, H., et al. "Aromatase in bone cell: association with osteoporosis in postmenopausal women." *J Steroid Biochem Mol Biol.* 1995; 53 (1-6): 165-74.

Obal, F., Jr., et al. "Inhibition of growth hormone-releasing factor suppresses both sleep and growth hormone secretion in the rat." *Brain Res.* 1991; 557 (1-2): 9-53.

Ohtsoka, A., et al. "Reduction of corticosterone-induced muscle proteolysis and growth retardation by a combined treatment with insulin, testosterone and high-protein-high-fat diet in rats." *NutrSci Vitaminol.* Tokyo. 1992; 38 (1): 83-92.

Oliva, A., et al. "Contribution of environmental factors to the risk of male infertility." *Hum Reprod.* 2001; 16 (8): 1768-76.

Opstad, P. K. "Androgenic hormones during prolonged physical stress, sleep energy deficiency." *J Clin Endocrinol Metab.* 1992; 74 (5): 1176-83.

Orden, I., et al. "Thyroxine in unextracted urine." *Acta Endocrinol (Copenh).* 1987; 114: 503-8.

Oventreich, N., et al. "Age changes and sex differences in serum DHEAs concentrations throughout adulthood." *J Clin Endocrinol Metab.* 1984; 59:551-55.

Overgaard, O., et al. "Effect of salcatonin given intranasally on bone mass and fracture rates in established osteoporosis: a dose-response study." *Br Med J.* 1992; 305: 556-61.

Peters, G. N., et al. "Estrogen replacement therapy after breast cancer: a 12-year follow-up." *Ann Surg Oncol.* 2001; 8 (10): 828-32.

Petridou, E., et al. "Pregnancy estrogens in relation to coffee and alcohol intake." *Ann Epidemiol.* 1992; 2 (3): 241-47.

Phillips, T. J., et al. "Hormonal effects on skin aging." *Clin Geriatr Med.* 2001; 17 (4): 661-72.

Picazo, O., et al. "Anti-anxiety effects of progesterone and some of its reduced metabolites: an evaluation using the burying behavior test." *Brain Res.* 1995; 680 (1-2): 135-41.

Porter, V R., et al. "Immune effects of hormone replacement therapy in post-menopausal women." *Exp Gerontol.* 2001; 36 (2): 311-26.

Rakic, Z., et al. "Testosterone treatment in men with erectile disorder and low levels of total testosterone in serum." *Arch Sex Behav.* 1997; 26 (5): 495-504.

Rao, M. S., et al. "Inhibition of spontaneous testicular Leydig cell tumor development in F-344 rats by dehydroepiandrosterone." *Cancer Lett.* 1992; 65 (2): 123-26.

Rebuffe-Scrive, M., et al. "Effect of testosterone on abdominal adipose tissue in men." *Int J Obes.* 1991; 15 (11): 791-95.

Regelson, W., et al. "DHEA the multifunctional steroid." *Annals NY Acad Sci.* 1994; 719: 564-75.

Reichlin, S., et al. "The role of stress in female reproductive dysfunction." *J Human Stress.* 1979; 5 (2): 38-45.

Reiter, R. "Protecting your heart." In *Melatonin: Breakthrough discoveries that can help you.* New York: Bantam Books, 1995; 106-22.

Reiter, R. J., et al. "A review of the evidence supporting melatonin's role as an antioxidant." *J Pineal Res.* 1995; 18 (1): 1-11.

Reiter, R. J., et al. "Melatonin and its relation to the immune system and inflammation." *Ann NY Acad Sci.* 2000; 917: 376-86.

Reiter, R. J., et al. Melatonin: the discoveries that can help you. New York: Bantam Books, 1995.

Reiter, W J., et al. "Dehydroepiandrosterone in the treatment of erectile dysfunction: a prospective, double-blind, randomized, placebo-controlled study." *Urology.* 1999; 53 (3): 590-94; discussion 594-95.

Reiter, W. J., et al. "Placebo-controlled dihydroepiandrosterone substitution in elderly men." *Gynakol Geburtshilfliche Rundsch.* 1999; 39 (4): 208-9.

Reiter, W. J., et al. "Serum dehydroepiandrosterone sulfate concentrations in men with erectile dysfunction." *Urology*. 2000; 55 (5): 755-58.

Reynard, J. M., et al. "Prostate-specific antigen and prognosis in patients with metastatic prostate cancer-a multivariable analysis of prostate cancer mortality. *Br J Urol*. 1995; 75 (4): 507-15.

Ribot, C., et al. "Bone mineral density and thyroid hormone therapy." *Clin Endocrinol (Oxf)*. 1990; 33 (2): 143-53.

Roberts, E. "Dehydroepiandrosterone (DHEA) and its sulfate (DHEAs) as neural facilitators: effects on brain tissue in culture and on memory in young and old mice. A cyclic GMP hypothesis of action of DHEA and DHEAs in nervous system and other tissues." In *The Biological Role of DHEA*, eds. W. Regelson and M. Kalimi. Berlin: Walter de Gruyter & Co., 1990; 13-42.

Roberts, E., et al. "Oral DHEA in multiple sclerosis: Results of a phase one, open study." *Dans: The Biological Role of DHEA*. Berlin: Walter de Gruyter, 1990; 81-93.

Robinzon, B., et al. "Should dehydroepiandrosterone replacement therapy be provided with glucocorticoids?" *Rheumatology (Oxf)*. 1999; 38 (6): 488-95.

Rojdmark, S., et al. "Effect of short-term fasting on nocturnal melatonin secretion in obesity." *Metabolism*. 1992; 41 (10): 1106-9.

Rollero, A., et al. "Relationship between cognitive function, growth hormone and insulin-like growth factor I plasma levels in aged subjects." *Neuropsychobiology*. 1998; 38 (2): 73-79.

Romagnoli, E., et al. "Effect of estrogen deficiency on IGF-I plasma levels: relationship with bone mineral density in perimenopausal women." *Calcif Tissue Int*. 1993; 53 (I): 1-6.

Rosano, G. M., et al. "Natural progesterone, but not medroxyprogesterone acetate, enhances the beneficial effect of estrogen on exercise-induced myocardial ischemia in postmenopausal women." *J Am Coll Cardiol*. 2000; 36 (7): 2154-59.

Rosen, T., et al. "Premature mortality due to cardiovascular disease in hypopituitarism." *Lancet*. 1990; 336: 285-88.

Rosenbaum, M., et al. "Effects of systemic growth hormone (GH) administration on regional adipose tissue in children with non-GH-deficient short stature." *J Clin Endocrinol Metab*. 1992; 75 (1): 151-56.

Rosenfeld, R. S., et al. "Metabolism and interconversion of dehydroisoandrosterone and dehydroisoandrosterone sulfate." *J Clin Endocrinol Metab*. 1972; 35 (2): 187-93.

Ross, D. S., "Hyperthyroidism, thyroid hormone therapy bone." *Thyroid*. 1994; 4 (3): 319-26.

Rozenberg, S., et al. "Age, steroids and bone mineral content." *Maturitas*. 1990;12:137-43.

Rudman, D., et al. "Impaired growth hormone secretion in the adult population. *J Clin Invest*. 1981; 67: 1361-69.

Russel Jones, D. L., et al. "The effect of growth hormone replacement on serum lipids, lipoproteins, apolipoproteins and cholesterol precursors in adult growth hormone deficient patients." *Clin Endocrinol (Oxf)*. 1994; 41 (3): 345-50.

Rutanen, E. M., et al. "Relationship between carbohydrate metabolism and serum insulin-like growth factor system in postmenopausal women: comparison of endometrial cancer patients with healthy controls." *J Clin Endocrinol Metab*. 1993; 77 (1): 199-204.

Salomen, F, et al. "Physiological role of growth hormone in adult life." In *Diagnosis and treatment of impaired growth hormone secretions*. ed. H. Flodh. Dorchester: Henry Ling Ltd.. 1987; 158-62.

Sambrook, P. N., et al. "Sex hormone status and osteoporosis in postmenopausal women with rheumatoid arthritis." *Arthritis Rheum*. 1988; 31 (8): 973-78.

Sambrook, P., et al. "Postmenopausal bone loss in rheumatoid arthritis: effect of estrogen and androgens." *J. Rheumatol*. 1992; 19 (3): 357-61.

Sandhu, G. S., et al. "Effect of L-thyroxine (LT4) and D-thyroxine (DT4) on cardiac function and high-energy phosphate metabolism: a 3 IP NMR study." *Magn Reson Med*. 1991; 18 (1): 237-43.

Sandstrom, N. J., et al. "Memory retention is modulated by acute estradiol and progesterone replacement."

Sandyk, R. "Estrogen's impact on cognitive functions in multiple sclerosis." *Int J Neurosci.* 1996; 86 (1-2): 23-31.

Sandyk, R., et al. "Is postmenopausal osteoporosis related to pineal gland functions?" *Int J Neurosci.* 1992; 62 (3-4): 215-25.

Sanmarti, A., et al. "Observational study in adult hypopituitary patients with untreated growth hormone deficiency (ODA study)." Socio-economic impact and health status. Collaborative ODA (Observational GH Deficiency in Adults) Group. *Eur J Endocrinol.* 1999; 141 (5): 481-89.

Sarrel, P. M. "Ovarian hormones and vaginal blood flow: using laser Doppler velocimetry to measure effects in a clinical trial of post-menopausal women." *Int J Impot Res.* 1998; 10 (Suppl 2): S91-93; discussion S98-101.

Sarrel, P. M. "Psychosexual effects of menopause: role of androgens." *Am J Obstet Gynecol.* 1999; 180 (3 Pt 2): S319-24.

Sarrel, P., et al. "Estrogen and estrogen-androgen replacement in postmenopausal women dissatisfied with estrogen-only therapy. Sexual behavior and neuroendocrine responses." *J Reprod Med.* 1998; 43 (10): 847-56.

Savuas, M., et al. "Type III collagen content in the skin of postmenopausal women receiving oestradiol and testosterone implants." *Br J Obstet Gynaecol.* 1993; 100 (2): 154-56.

Scarabin, P. Y., et al. "Effects of oral and transdermal estrogen/progesterone regimens on blood coagulation and fibrinolysis in postmenopausal women." A randomized controlled trial. *Arterioscler Thromb Vasc Biol.* 1997; 17 (11): 3071-78.

Schaeffer, M. A., et al. "Adrenal cortisol response to stress at Three Mile Island." *Psychosom Med.* 1984; 46 (3): 227.

Schatzl, G., et al. "Endocrine patterns in patients with benign and malignant prostatic diseases." *Prostate.* 2000; 44 (3): 219-24.

Schatzl, G., et al. "Endocrine status in elderly men with lower urinary tract symptoms: correlation of age, hormonal status lower urinary tract function. The Prostate Study Group of the Austrian Society of Urology." *Urology.* 2000; 55 (3): 397-402.

Schiavi, R. C., et al. "Pituitary-gonadal function during sleep in healthy aging men." *Psychoneuroendocrinology.* 1992; 17 (6): 599-609.

Schlaghecke, R., et al. "Effects of glucocorticoids in rheumatoid arthritis. Diminished glucocorticoid receptors do not result in glucocorticoid resistance." *Arthritis Rheum.* 1994; 37 (8): 1127-31.

Schmitt, T, et al. "Unresponsiveness to exogenesis TSH in obesity." *Int J. Obesity.* 1977; 1: 185-90.

Schultz, B. M., et al. "Iron deficiency in the elderly." *Baillieres Clin. Haenatole.* 1987; 291-313.

Schwartz, S. B. S. "The relationship of thyroid deficiency to cancer: a 50-year retrospective study." *J IAPM* 1977; VI (1): 9-2 1.

Seeger, H., et al. "Effect of medroxyprogesterone acetate and norethisterone on serumstimulated and estradiol-inhibited proliferation of human coronary artery smooth muscle cells." *Menopause.* 2001; 8 (1): 5-9.

Seidman SN, Testosterone and depression in aging men. Walsh BT Am J Geriatr Psychiatry 1999 Winter;7(1)18-33

Sekiguchi, R., et al. "Analysis of the influence of vasopressin neuropeptides on social memory of rats." *Eur Neuropsychopharmacol.* 1991; 2: 123-26.

Shabsigh, R. "The effects of testosterone on the cavernous tissue and erectile function." *World J Urol.* 1997; 15 (1): 21-26.

Shapiro, J., et al. "Testosterone and other anabolic steroids as cardiovascular drugs." *Am J Ther.* 1999; 6 (3): 167-74.

Shelton, B. K. "Hypothyroidism in cancer patients." *Nurse Pract Forum.* 1998; 9 (3): 185-91.

Sherwin, B. B. "Can estrogen keep you smart? Evidence from clinical studies." *J Psychiatry Neurosci.* 1999; 24 (4): 315-21.

Sherwin, B. B. "Estrogen and/or androgen replacement therapy and cognitive functioning in surgically menopausal women." *Psychoneuroendocrinology.* 1988; 13 (4): 345-57.

Shuster, J., et al. "The influence of age and sex on skin thickness, skin collagen and density." *Br J Dermatol*. 1975; 93: 639-43.

Simon, D., Preziosi, P., Barrett-Connor, E., Roger, M., Saint Paul, M., Nahoul, K., Papoz, L. The influence of aging on plasma sex hormones in men: the Telecom Study. *Am. J. Epidemiol.* 1992 Apr 1; 135(7): 783-91.

Simon, J. A., et al. "Safety profile: transdermal testosterone treatment of women after oophorectomy." *Obstet Gynecol*. 2001; 97 (4 Suppl 1): S10-S11.

Sipila, S., et al. "Effects of hormone replacement therapy and high-impact physical exercise on skeletal muscle in post-menopausal women: a randomized placebo-controlled study." *Clin Sci (Lond)*. 2001; 101 (2): 147-57.

Slocumb, C. H., "Cortisone and related steroids in the treatment of rheumatoid arthritis." *Med Clin North Am*. 1961; 45: 1209-18.

Smadel, J. E., et al. "Treatment of typhoid fever; combined therapy with cortisone and chloramphenicol." *Ann Intern Med*. 1951; 34: 1-9.

Smith, J. C., et al. "The effects of induced hypogonadism on arterial stiffness, body composition metabolic parameters in males with prostate cancer." *J Clin Endocrinol Metab*. 2001; 86 (9): 4261-67.

Smith, Y R., et al. "Long-term estrogen replacement is associated with improved nonverbal memory and attentional measures in postmenopausal women." *Fertil Steril*. 2001; 76 (6): 1101-7.

Snyder, P. J., et al. "Effects of testosterone replacement in hypogonadal men." *J Clin Endocrinol Metab*. 2000; 85 (8): 2670-77.

Sorensen, M. B., et al. "Obesity and sarcopenia after menopause are reversed by sex hormone replacement therapy." *Obes Res*. 2001; 9 (10): 622-26.

Stabler, B. "Impact of growth hormone (GH) therapy on quality of life along the lifespan of GHtreated patients." *Horm Res*. 2001; 56 Suppl 1: 55-58.

Stall, G. M., et al. "Accelerated bone loss in hypothyroid patients over treated with L-thyroxine." *Ann Intern Med*. 1990; 113 (4): 265-69.

Stampfer, M. J., et al. "Postmenopausal estrogen therapy and cardiovascular disease. Ten-year follow-up from the Nurses' Health study." *New Engl J Med*. 1991;325:756-62.

Stein, D. G. "Brain damage, sex hormones and recovery: a new role for progesterone and estrogen?" *Trends Neurosci*. 2001; 24 (7): 386-91.

Straub, R. H., et al. "Replacement therapy with DHEA plus corticosteroids in patients with chronic inflammatory diseases-substitutes of adrenal and sex hormones." *Z Rheumatol*. 2000; 59 (Suppl 2): II/108-18.

Taelman, P., et al. "Reduced forearm bone mineral content and biochemical evidence of increased bone turnover in women with euthyroid goitre treated with thyroid hormone." *Clin Endocrinol (Oxf)*. 1990; 33 (1): 107-17.

Taggart, H. M., et al. "Deficient calcitonin response to calcium stimulation in postmenopausal osteoporosis." *Lancet*. 1982; 1: 475-78.

Tan, R. S. "Memory loss as a reported symptom of andropause." *Arch Androl*. 2001; 47 (3): 185-89.

Tan, R. S., et al. "The andropause and memory loss: is there a link between androgen decline and dementia in the aging male?" Tannirandorn, P., et al. "Drug-induced bone loss." *Osteoporos Int*. 2000; 11 (8): 637-59. Review.

Tenover, J.S., Effects of testosterone supplementation in the aging male. *J. Clin. Endocrinol. Metab*. 1992; 75(4): 1092-8.

Terzolo, M., et al. "Effects of long-term, low-dose, time-specified melatonin administration on endocrine and cardiovascular variables in adult men." *J Pineal Res*. 1990; 9 (2): 113-24.

Thomas, R., et al. "Thyroid disease and reproductive function: a review." *Obstet Gynecol*. 1987; 70: 789.

Tomanek, R. J., et al. "Initiation of cardiac hypertrophy in response to thyroxin is not limited by age." *Am J Physiol*. 1993; 264 (4 Pt 2): H1041-47.

Tomer, Y., et al. "Infection, thyroid disease autoimmunity." *Endocr Rev.* 1993; 14 (1): 107-20.

Twycross, R. "The risks and benefits of corticosteroids in advanced cancer." *Drug Saf.* 1994; 11 (3): 163-78.

Tymchuk, C. N., et al. "Evidence of an inhibitory effect of diet and exercise on prostate cancer cell growth." *J Urol.* 2001; 166 (3): 1185-89.

Vallee, M., et al. "Role of pregnenolone, dehydroepiandrosterone and their sulfate esters on learning and memory in cognitive aging." *Brain Res Rev.* 2001; 37 (1-3): 301-12.

Van Cauter, E., et al. "Demonstration of rapid light-induced advances and delays of the human circadian clock using hormonal phase markers." *Am J Physiol.* 1994; 266 (6, part 1): E953-63.

Van Goozen, Z. H., et al. "Psychoendocrinological assessment of the menstrual cycle: the relationship between hormones, sexuality mood." *Arch Sex Behav.* 1997; 26 (4): 359-82.

Van Vollenhoven, R. F., et al. "An open study of DHEA in SLE." *Arthritis Rheum.* 1994; 37 (9): 1305-12.

Van Weerden, W. M., et al. "Effect of adrenal androgens on the transplantable human prostate tumor." *Endocrinology.* 1992; 131 (6): 2909-13.

Vandenbroucke, J. P., et al. "Noncontraceptive hormones and rheumatoid arthritis in perimenopausal and postmenopausal women." *JAMA.* 1986; 255 (10): 1299-1303.

Vander Veen, E. A., et al. "Growth hormone (replacement) therapy in adults: bone and calcium metabolism." *Horm Res.* 1990; 33 (Suppl 4): 65-68.

Vandewighe, M., et al. "Short- and long-term effects of growth hormone treatment on bone turnover and bone mineral content in adult growth hormone deficient males." *Clin Endocrinol (Oxf).* 1993; 39 (4): 409-15.

Villareal, D. T., et al. "Effects of DHEA replacement on bone mineral density and body composition in elderly women and men." *Clin Endocrinol (Oxf).* 2000; 53 (5): 561-68.

Volek, J. S., et al. "Testosterone and cortisol in relationship to dietary nutrients and resistance exercise." *J Appl Physiol.* 1997; 82 (1): 49-54.

Vollestad, N. K., et al. "Biochemical correlates with fatigue." *Eur J Appl Physiol.* 1988; 57: 336-47.

Waldhauser, G., et al. "Alterations in nocturnal serum melatonin levels in humans with growth and aging." *J Clin Endocrinol Metab.* 1988; 66: 648-52.

Walker, I. D., et al. "Effect of anabolic steroids on plasma antithrombin III." *Thrombos Diathes Haemorrh (Stuttg).* 1975; 34: 106.

Wallgren, P., et al. "Influence of experimentally induced endogenous production of cortisol on the immune capacity in swine." *Vet Immunol Immunopathol.* 1994; 42 (3-4): 301-16.

Wallymahmed, M. E., et al. "The quality of life of adults with growth hormone deficiency: comparison with diabetic patients and control subjects." *Clin Endocrinol (Oxf).* 1999; 51 (3): 333-38.

Wang, C., et al. "Transdermal testosterone gel improves sexual function, mood, muscle strength body composition parameters in hypogonadal men." *J Clin Endocrinol Metab.* 2000; 85 (8): 2839-53.

Watkins, P. J., "Clinical Presentation: why is diabetes so often missed?" In *ABC of Diabetes.* 4th ed. London: BMJ Publishing Group, 1998; 6-19.

Watts, N. B., et al. "Comparison of oral estrogens and estrogens plus androgen on bone mineral density, menopausal symptoms lipid-lipoprotein profiles in surgical menopause." *Obstet Gynecol.* 1995; 85 (4): 529-37.

Weaver, J. U., et al. "The effect of growth hormone replacement on cortisol metabolism and glucocorticoid sensitivity in hypopituitary adults." *Clin Endocrinol (Oxf).* 1994; 41 (5): 639-48.

Weitzman, S., et al. "Clinical trial design in studies of corticosteroids in bacterial infections." *Ann Intern Med.* 1974; 81: 36-42.

Werner, A. A. "The male climacteric." *JAMA.* 1946; 132 (4): 188-94.

Wheeler, G. D., et al. "Endurance training decreases serum testosterone levels in men without change in LH pulsatile release." *J Clin Endocrinol Metab.* 1991; 72: 422-29.

Wiener, B., et al. "Age; sex and serum thyrotropin concentrations in primary hypothyroidism." *Acta Endocrinol Copenh.* 1991; 124 (4): 364-69.

Wimalawansa, S. J., et al. "The effect of percutaneous oestradiol and low dose human calcitonin on postmenopausal vertebral bone loss." *Osteoporosis.* 1987; 528-32.

Wingo, P. A., et al. "The risk of breast cancer in postmenopausal women who have used estrogen replacement therapy." (Published erratum appears in JAMA. 1987; 257 [18]: 2438.) *JAMA.* 1987; 257 (2): 209-15.

Wolden-Hanson, T., et al. "Daily melatonin administration to middle-aged male rats suppresses body weight, intraabdominal adiposity plasma leptin and insulin independent of food intake and total body fat." *Endocrinology.* 2000; 141 (2): 487-97.

Wolf, D. A., et al. "Synthetic androgens suppress the transformed phenotype in human prostate carcinoma cell line LNCaP." *Br J Cancer.* 1991; 64 (1): 47-53.

Wolf, O. T., et al. "Effects of a two-week physiological dehydroepiandrosterone substitution on cognitive performance and well-being in healthy elderly women and men." *J Clin Endocrinol Metab.* 1997; 82 (7): 2363-67.

Wolkowitz, U. M., et al. "Antidepressant and cognition-enhancing effects of DHEA in major depression." *Ann NY Acad Sci.* 1995; 774: 337-39.

Wortsmann, J., et al. "Abnormal testicular function in men with primary hypothyroidism." *Am J Med.* 1987; 82: 207.

Wright J.V, MD & Morgenthaler J. "Natural Hormone Replacement" - Smart Publications 1997

Wuster, C., et al. "Decreased serum levels on insulin-like growth factors and IGF binding protein 3 in osteoporosis." *J Intern Med.* 1993; 234 (3): 249-55.

Wuster, C., et al. "Increased prevalence of osteoporosis and arteriosclerosis in conventionally substituted anterior pituitary insufficiency: need for additional growth hormone substitution." *Klin Wochenschr.* 1991; 18, 69 (16): 769-73.

Yang, R., et al. "Growth hormone improves cardiac performances in experimental heart failure." *Circulation.* 1995; 92 (2): 262-67.

Zhdanova, I. V., et al. "Sleep-inducing effects of low doses of melatonin ingested in the evening." *Clin Pharmacol. Ther.* 1995; 57 (5): 552-58.

Zumoff, B., et al. "Sex differences in twenty-four-hour mean plasma concentrations of DHEA and DHEAS and the DHEA to DHEAs ratio in normal adults." *J Clin Endocrinol Metab.* 1980; 51 (2): 330-33.

Van den Beld, A. W., et al. "Measures of bioavailable serum testosterone and estradiol and their relationships with muscle strength, bone density body composition in elderly men." *J Clin Endocrinol Metab.* 2000; 85 (9): 3276-82.

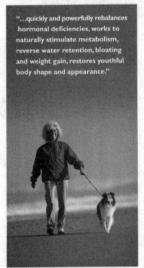

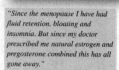
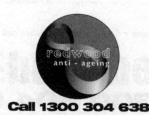

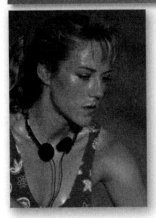
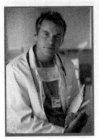
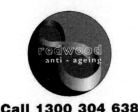